WAY

The Columbia Presbyterian Osteoarthritis Handbook

FUNDS TO PURCHASE
THIS BOOK WERE
PROVIDED BY A
40TH ANNIVERSARY GRANT
FROM THE
FOELLINGER FOUNDATION.

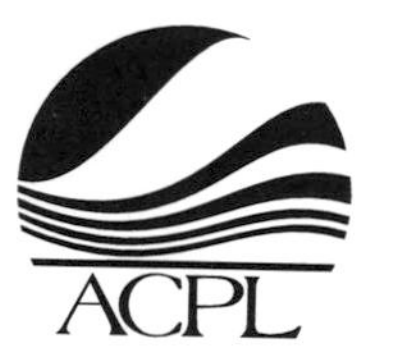

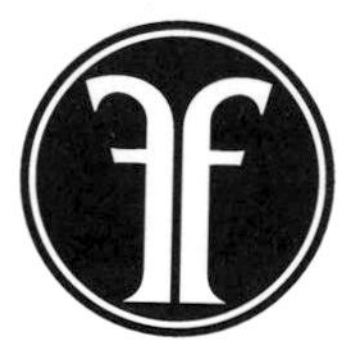

The Columbia Presbyterian Osteoarthritis Handbook

The Complete Guide to the Most Common Form of Arthritis

RONALD P. GRELSAMER, M.D.,
AND SUZANNE LOEBL,
Editors

Macmillan • USA

MACMILLAN
A Simon & Schuster Macmillan Company
1633 Broadway
New York, NY 10019-6785

Library of Congress Cataloging-in-Publication Data
The Columbia Presbyterian osteoarthritis handbook : the complete guide to the most common form of arthritis / Ronald P. Grelsamer, M.D., and Suzanne Loebl, editors.
p. cm.
Includes index.
ISBN 0-02-861904-8
1. Osteoarthritis—Popular works. I. Grelsamer, Ronald P. II. Loebl, Suzanne.
RC931.067C65 1996
616.7'223—dc20 95-24782
CIP

Illustrations by Caroline Meinstein

Manufactured in the United States of America
10 9 8 7 6 5 4 3 2 1

This book is not intended as a substitute for medical advice of physicians. The reader should regularly consult a physician in matters relating to his or her health and particularly with respect to any symptoms that might require diagnosis or medical attention.

Dedication

To my grandchildren: Ana, Naomi, and Sean Gordon-Loebl.

—SL

To my parents. To my wife, Sharon, and my children, Dominique and Marc. To my patients past, present, and future, May you always be informed consumers.

—RPG

Acknowledgments

The writing of *The Columbia Presbyterian Osteoarthritis Handbook* was a team effort. It is the hope of the editors and contributors that those who read this book will live more comfortably and participate more fully and knowledgeably in decisions involving their care and surgical options.

Any medical self-help book draws on works written by others in the same field. This is particularly true of a reference work. The editors consulted numerous textbooks in rheumatology and orthopedics as well as patient education publications developed by the Arthritis Foundation and the American Academy of Orthopedic Surgeons.

The editors want specifically to thank the following:

The Arthritis Foundation for their excellent publications, including their magazine, *Arthritis Today*, and their *Primer on Rheumatic Diseases*. The first offered inspiration, the second hard facts. We also want to thank the Foundation for permission to reproduce their "Range of Motion Exercises." The staff of the Foundation was helpful whenever the need arose. Special thanks go to Dorothy Goldstein of the New York Chapter of the Arthritis Foundation, who arranged the visit to the Aquatic Exercise Program at the New York City YWCA.

Thanks are also due to the following:

David Ginsberg, Deputy to the President of Presbyterian Hospital, without whom the book would never have been developed.

Judy H. Loebl, physical therapist, who served as a general advisor on musculoskeletal problems.

J. Frank Hatch, another physical therapist, for his advice.

Patrician Reagan Argiro, who read the entire manuscript throughout various stages and provided constructive criticism. Her enthusiasm and faith in the project were crucial to the completion of the book.

The Center for Biomedical Communication for the photograph of the arthroscope; Sergio A. Jimenez, M.D., for the illustration of collagen fibers in various tissues; and the Metropolitan Life Insurance Company of America for the Table of the Ideal Body Weights.

Employees of Columbia Presbyterian, especially the staff of the operating rooms; Sandra Walsh, director of the Patients Relations Department; Shelly Warwick, librarian of the Russel A. Hibbs Memorial Library; and Donna McCarthy, Director of Admittance at Milstein Hospital.

Our editor, Nancy Cooperman, who has given us the benefit of her skill and did a superb job editing the book.

Finally, our warmest thanks go to the many patients who shared their private experiences and feelings with the authors, thereby making this book more personal and readable.

Contributors

Louis U. Bigliani, M.D.
Chief, The Shoulder Service
Professor of Orthopedic Surgery
The Columbia Presbyterian Medical Center

Harold M. Dick, M.D.
Director, New York Orthopedic Hospital
The Columbia Presbyterian Medical Center

Therese Ann Franzese, M.S., R.D.
Assistant Professor
Department of Clinical Nutrition
New York Institute of Technology

Ronald P. Grelsamer, M.D.
Chief, Hip and Knee Reconstruction
Maimonides Medical Center
Staff Orthopedic Surgeon
Hospital for Joint Diseases and Beth Israel North

Terrence F. O'Halloran, M.S., P.T.
Senior Physical Therapist and Clinical Instructor
College of Physicians and Surgeons, Columbia University

Suzanne Loebl
Vice-Chair
Columbia Presbyterian Community Health Council

Stanley Myers, M.D.
A. David Gurewitsch Professor of Clinical Rehabilitation Medicine
College of Physicians and Surgeons, Columbia University

Katherine G. Nickerson, M.D.
Assistant Clinical Professor of Medicine
College of Physicians and Surgeons, Columbia University

Anthony Ratcliffe, Ph.D.
Associate Professor of Orthopedic Biochemistry
College of Physicians and Surgeons, Columbia University

Mark Weidenbaum, M.D.
Associate Professor of Clinical Orthopedic Surgery
College of Physicians and Surgeons, Columbia University

Contents

Introduction

Who Should Read This Book

All forms of arthritis, including osteoarthritis, are diseases that require informed self-care. To put it differently: The more you know about your disease, and the better you understand the purpose of the prescribed medications and exercises, the more you will be able to

- maintain your normal lifestyle
- live without pain
- follow doctors' orders intelligently
- take part in the decision-making process
- remain in charge of your own life

Patient self-empowerment is the principal purpose of *The Columbia Presbyterian Osteoarthritis Handbook.*

This book is written by staff members of Columbia Presbyterian Medical Center.

The editors of this book are Ronald P. Grelsamer, M.D., and Suzanne Loebl. Dr. Grelsamer is a physician specializing in musculoskeletal disorders and an orthopedic surgeon concentrating on the surgery of the hips and knees. Suzanne Loebl is a former science editor of the Arthritis Foundation and a victim of osteoarthritis. This book is for people suffering from osteoarthritis and their families, as well as for those undergoing joint replacement and back surgery as treatment for other ailments.

Who Has Osteoarthritis?

It is said that if you live long enough you will develop arthritis. This fortunately is not true. Only about 10 percent of the population suffer from arthritis severe enough to require medical care.

You may know that *arthritis* is the family name of about one hundred assorted diseases. Their common bond is joint pain; their other symptoms and their causes are highly varied. The arthritides—plural of arthritis and one family name for this group of diseases—include rheumatoid arthritis (a crippling form of the disease related to a malfunction of the immune system), gout (a metabolic disorder), systemic lupus erythematosus, juvenile rheumatoid arthritis, dermatomyositis, Reiter's syndrome, and many others. According to the National Arthritis Data Workgroup, "Arthritis and other disorders of the musculoskeletal system comprise the most frequently reported cause of impairment affecting the adult population of the United States." Specific complaints include acute and chronic symptoms of joint swelling, limitation of motion, pain upon motion, or backaches.

This book concerns itself only with osteoarthritis (OA), by far the most common form of the disease, and the one that most affects older persons. Since America is graying, osteoarthritis is getting more and more common.

Exact figures on how many people suffer from osteoarthritis are difficult to come by. A definite diagnosis involves X-ray demonstration of alteration of the structure of the joint. Yet many people with such radiographic evidence do not have any discomfort. According to the latest figures of the National Center for Health Statistics, osteoarthritis affects *15.8 million* persons severely enough to require medical care.

In addition there are millions of sufferers who do not go to the doctor because they feel that "there is nothing medicine can do about arthritis." Others, with less severe disease, successfully manage on their own.

A growing number of younger people develop osteoarthritis because of an athletic or other traumatic injury or developmental malalignment of their musculoskeletal system. For them, timely treatment, joint protection, and judiciously prescribed exercises often prevent or arrest progression of the disease.

WHAT IS OSTEOARTHRITIS?

Let us begin with the following reassurances for those of you suffering from osteoarthritis:

- Osteoarthritis does not cripple (twist your body into a pretzel) or disfigure. The disease affects individual joints. Even when severe, osteoarthritis is limited to the joints and will not affect your internal organs—the liver, heart, lungs, or kidneys.
- For most patients medical management with exercise, medication, splints, rest, heat, and similar measures is highly successful.
- Persons developing osteoarthritis during the closing years of the twentieth century are very fortunate. If medical management fails, most patients have a surgical option. During recent decades orthopedic surgery has made tremendous strides. Today most joints—and even the back—can be repaired and reconstructed.

The growing importancc of orthopcdic surgery in the United States is best illustrated by the number of operations performed annually. According to the National Center for Health Statistics, in 1991 there were

117,000 total hip replacements, 90,000 partial hip replacements, and 25,000 hip revisions.

160,000 total knee replacements and 17,000 revisions.

4,000 total shoulder replacements and 2,000 partial shoulder replacements.

140,000 spinal fusions and 306,000 intervertebral disk excisions or destructions.

The Columbia Presbyterian Osteoarthritis Handbook will walk you through the total joint replacement operations used for patients suffering from osteoarthritis. This portion of the *Handbook* is also useful for anyone undergoing this type of surgery for reasons other than osteoarthritis.

YOUR MEDICAL TEAM

Good medical care for osteoarthritis usually requires several members of a health care team, including

- physicians
- orthopedic surgeons
- physical therapists
- pharmacists
- occupational therapists
- rehabilitation specialists
- dietitians

In the *The Columbia Presbyterian Osteoarthritis Handbook:*

Harold M. Dick, M.D., Director of New York Orthopedic Hospital, reviews general facts about osteoarthritis and introduces you to your medical team.

Katherine Nickerson, M.D., masterminds and coordinates your medical care. She reviews commonly used diagnostic tests for osteoarthritis and describes the overall treatment program.

Anthony Ratcliffe, Ph.D., an authority on cartilage, the soft, gristlelike material that is the target of osteoarthritis, reviews the overall structure of joints and explains in what way these are affected by osteoarthritic disease processes. Dr. Ratcliffe also speculates about scientific advances that may improve medical treatment.

Ronald P. Grelsamer, M.D., reviews the many medications used for osteoarthritis.

Terrence O'Halloran, M.S., P.T., one of Columbia Presbyterian's senior physical therapists of acute care, teaches you how to exercise your joints cautiously, so that you may prevent further joint damage.

Stanley Myers, M.D., a rehabilitation specialist, describes nonpharmacological methods of pain relief.

Therese Ann Franzese, M.S., R.D., a staff nutritionist, talks about food and arthritis.

Suzanne Loebl, coauthor, contributes her double expertise as a longtime science editor of the Arthritis Foundation and as an osteoarthritis patient.

The surgical interventions used in the treatment of osteoarthritis are reviewed by staff members of the Department of Orthopedic Surgery at

Columbia Presbyterian Medical Center, the successor of the New York Orthopedic Hospital (NYOH) founded by Dr. George Fayette Taylor in 1866. Theodore Roosevelt Sr., father of the president, was the driving force behind the effort. Dr. Taylor had successfully treated Roosevelt's daughter Anna for spinal disease. Her father, together with four friends, wanted to provide orthopedic care for New York's poor children.

A small brownstone housed the original New York Orthopedic Dispensary at 1299 Broadway. The institution moved to larger quarters in 1873, and to a quite impressive complex at 420 East Fifty-ninth Street in 1916. The NYOH established a link with Columbia University in 1918 and became formally affiliated with Columbia Presbyterian in 1945. It moved to the medical center campus in 1950.

For 128 years the NYOH provided New Yorkers with superior orthopedic care. Not surprisingly, *U.S. News and World Report* ranked the Department of Orthopedic Surgery at Columbia Presbyterian Medical Center among the best in the country.

Innovation was always one of the hallmarks of the NYOH approach. Forty years ago, in 1956, the hospital established the Orthopedic Research Laboratory now staffed by forty-eight researchers. The laboratory played a leading role in the development of prostheses of the hip, shoulder, and knee. Patients suffering from osteoarthritis and traumatic joint injury now are major beneficiaries of the diligent work of these researchers.

Leading orthopedists have governed NYOH during its 125-year history. Today the clinical faculty of twenty-two physicians is headed by **Harold M. Dick, M.D.,** who specializes in musculoskeletal tumor surgery in children and adults. Trained at Columbia Presbyterian and a member of its faculty ever since, Dr. Dick assumed the directorship in 1984. Under his leadership the hospital enlarged its involvement in biotechnology and bioengineering and expanded its trauma program to include the Harlem Hospital Center and the Helen Hayes Hospital and Medical Center.

It is a great credit to the institution that most of the physicians on the staff of the Department of Orthopedics trained at Columbia University Medical School. In addition to caring for their own patients, staff members are orthopedic consultants for the New York Yankees.

The following orthopedic surgeons contributed chapters to *The Columbia Presbyterian Osteoarthritis Handbook:*

The general editor, **Ronald P. Grelsamer, M.D.,** helps you decide if and when you should have surgery, tells you how to prepare for your hospital stay, and reviews such novel practices as autologous blood transfusion and same-day surgery.

Dr. Grelsamer also reviews osteoarthritis of the lower extremities (hips, knee, and feet). He lets you watch over his shoulder while he reconstructs a hip and a knee.

Back pain is one of America's major health problems. **Mark Weidenbaum, M.D.,** reviews the medical and surgical treatment of the common osteoarthritic changes of the back.

Louis Bigliani, M.D., discusses the shoulder. Dr. Bigliani's patients include victims of osteoarthritis as well as leading musicians and sports figures who have shoulder complaints that are a kind of "occupational hazard."

Robert Strauch, M.D., and the occupational therapist **Robin Akdeniz** explore osteoarthritic hands and elbows.

Each surgical chapter includes an in-depth discussion of the anatomy and function of particular joints or group of joints. This knowledge will prove valuable to all those whose shoulders, knees, hips, or hands are affected by disease or trauma, whether they need surgery or not.

Health care providers are not the only teachers you'll meet in *The Columbia Presbyterian Osteoarthritis Handbook.* Realizing that much helpful information comes from people who have experienced similar medical problems, your editors talked to scores of medical and surgical patients suffering from osteoarthritis. This book incorporates their comments and personal experiences with treatments and surgical procedures.

Medicine today is much better than it used to be, but it is also much less friendly. Relations between doctor and patient can become downright hostile. This book reviews practical ways of building a lasting, good relationship with your physicians.

Medical care has become so expensive that only a very few can pay for it out of their own pocket. Medical reimbursements by Medicare and Blue Cross–Blue Shield are now so complex that hospitals have specialists dealing with such "entitlements." In Appendix II of this book, your editors explore ways to address your special concerns about hospital policies and the cost of your treatment.

How to Use This Book

The authors hope that *The Columbia Presbyterian Osteoarthritis Handbook* will become a trusted companion; that as you read it you will learn how to participate in your own care and remain as pain-free and active as you can. You have to. Life expectancy is increasing. By and large, patients suffering from osteoarthritis are a healthy lot. Learning to deal with their osteoarthritis intelligently will make their future years more enjoyable.

This book is subdivided into two parts:

Part I explains the nature of the disease and presents an overview of medical treatments (diagnosis, drug therapy, exercise, rest, pain relief, diet).

Part II explores criteria to consider when contemplating joint surgery. Thereafter it details the surgical reconstruction of the individual joints. Appendix I answers the most frequently asked questions about osteoarthritis. Appendix II takes a fresh look at the treatment of osteoarthritis for the updated edition of this book. Appendix III lists the currently available nonsteroidal anti-inflammatory drugs (NSAIDS). The book concludes with a glossary of medical terms commonly used during arthritis care.

◆ PART ◆ I

General Management of Osteoarthritis

◆ CHAPTER ◆

1

Five Patients

Naomi B.

Naomi was proud and relieved. She watched as 190 young men and women marched up to receive their diplomas from the dean of the University of California Berkeley Business School. Her son was among the graduates. After a five-week European vacation, David would be an account executive at the American Telephone and Telegraph Company.

But all was not well with Naomi. A nagging pain radiated from her upper abdomen to her feet. The pain was moderate, but constant and nagging. It was much worse in the evening than in the morning, but it never went away completely. What was it? Cancer? A bad back? Too much tension? Arthritis?

When she returned from the graduation, Naomi went to see her family physician, who told her to get an X ray. One look at the X ray convinced the doctor that Naomi suffered from osteoarthritis of the hip. The arthritis was mild, the doctor told her, adding that it would be years before she had real trouble. But Naomi was shocked and worried. Wasn't forty-five much too young an age at which to have osteoarthritis?

Claude B.

Claude B. raced through the powdery snow in Vail. Barely halting for a deep breath after the downhill run, he headed for the chairlift. In

January the days were short, and he wanted to get the most out of his trip to Colorado. Watching him, nobody would believe that Claude is seventy-one years old, had a total hip replacement eight years ago, a four-vessel coronary bypass six years ago, and a total knee replacement nine months ago.

The physicians who keep Claude in "working order" admire his athletic performance. His surgeons, however, disapprove of his skiing: "What if he injures one of his new joints," says one of them. "His new hip and his new knee are excellent. They nevertheless are breakable mechanical devices that should not be overstressed. It is very difficult to reconstruct a joint the first time around. It is even trickier to repair it when it breaks or fails. Moreover, the operation is seldom as successful."

Claude had injured his knee severely in 1941, while serving in the U.S. ski-troops during World War II. "You'll never ski again," the army surgeon said after he fixed Claude's knee. Fifty years ago there were no arthroscopes and other techniques that orthopedists use today, and Claude's recovery was very slow. He used crutches to begin with, then a cane. But he swam and hiked and within a few years started to ski again—a little at first, then as often as he could. Sure, the knee troubled him at times, but Claude just did not pay any attention.

In May 1984 Claude's joints acted up. The trouble started suddenly. As Claude was taking a four-mile stroll, he felt such a sharp pain in his groin that he simply could not continue walking. He flagged down a car, which took him back home.

There the pain vanished, but soon came back. Claude tried to ignore it and go on with life as usual. After four weeks of intermittent discomfort, he consulted a physical therapist, who said it was "a typical athlete's irritation" and prescribed heat therapy and exercises.

The pain persisted. A doctor diagnosed "a touch of osteoarthritis of the hip" and recommended a cane and rest. The pain escalated. Claude could not sleep at night. He would get up, sit in a chair for a bit, then lie down and sleep a bit more until the pain woke him again. Claude recalls that the pain was so bad that he considered suicide. Instead he visited many doctors and alternative health care providers. They prescribed relaxation, aspirin, and acupuncture.

The pain continued to poison his life. Less than six months after the first symptom, Claude decided to undergo a total hip replacement. It was successful, but two years later Claude was back at the hospital for a coronary bypass operation.

Claude recovered. He gardened, hiked, and skied, but his troubles were not over. Remember the knee? In 1991, fifty years after the original injury, it finally gave up. An X-ray showed that the cartilage was all gone and brittle bone now rubbed on brittle bone. Small pieces of bone broke off and fell into the joint cavity, causing intense inflammation. Spells of acute pain followed, lasting about twenty-four hours, then abated. But gradually the episodes occurred more and more often. "Enough," said Claude, "I need a new knee."

BERNICE S.

As she combed her hair, Bernice S., a real-estate agent, noticed that her hands "looked awfully old, like those of a very old woman." When she was younger, Bernice loved her small, dainty hands with their well-manicured nails. Rings were her favorite pieces of jewelry. Now her fingers looked old and crooked.

Bernice explained that "it all started about twenty years ago, when the pinkie on my left hand just did not work right, and it hurt when I bumped it. I just did not pay very much attention.

"Then, one day when I wanted to take off my wedding band it simply would not come off. I tried and tried. Finally I went to a jeweler, who cut it off.

"Soon all my fingers gave me trouble. One or two finger joints would become painful for weeks or months at a time. Then the joint would calm down, but the finger would never work quite the same again.

"I was getting awfully clumsy. Ten or twelve years ago I kept dropping plates and could not pick up pots. Writing became tiresome and sewing impossible. Now I seem to have adjusted to my osteoarthritic fingers. I slice and peel vegetables and have learned how to lift plates and pots. I cannot hold anything in my hand for too long. After a while I just drop whatever I am holding. When I have to carry something, I must support it with my whole arm.

"I do have osteoarthritis elsewhere, especially in my neck, but I manage to live with that, too. I sleep with a chiro-pillow, which is cut out where the neck fits. About two years ago I changed my diet. I cut out nightshade vegetables, like white potatoes and tomatoes. I don't know whether that helped. I feel OK and continue to sell houses. I still don't wear my rings. Though I had them enlarged, they just don't look nice on my big lumpy fingers," she said with a resigned sigh.

ANDREA L.

Lights dim in a small auditorium. The chatter and the coughing of the audience fade. The conductor enters. After a welcoming applause, the orchestra starts up. The violin, played by Andrea L., leads the way. Andrea L. is playing for the first time after months of inactivity.

Andrea L., now fifty-four, took up the violin as a child. As a teenager she also seriously studied piano and ballet. Eventually her mother insisted that Andrea choose one art form, arguing that she could not afford lessons for all three. The violin won out.

Like other professional musicians Andrea practiced all the time, especially after she was admitted to Juilliard, one of the top music conservatories in America. She listened to her teachers, played intensely for hours.

"A violin is for expressing emotion," Andrea explains. "Playing sometimes causes tension and pain."

In 1960 Andrea married and delightedly took care of her husband and three boys. Music, for a very short time, played "second fiddle." She continued to practice and perform occasionally.

Then in 1971, when she was thirty-three, she set her sights on becoming a member of the Colonial Symphony Orchestra in Madison, New Jersey. She practiced at least four to five hours a day. Her talent and diligence paid off, and that year she was admitted as an orchestra member. She often performed solo parts with the orchestra and gave solo and chamber music recitals and benefits.

Andrea's fulfilling life lasted for about fifteen years; then her shoulder started hurting. For a very long time Andrea tried to ignore the pain. She tried simple remedies: different-size pads to rest her violin on her shoulder; holding her violin differently; practicing less. She took hot baths after playing for a long time.

"I never thought of my shoulder problem as being an occupational hazard," she says now.

Eventually the pain was so bad that Andrea sought medical advice. She went to see several physical therapists, an osteopath, and family physicians. X rays were taken. Andrea faithfully performed the prescribed therapeutic exercises, took anti-inflammatory drugs and corticosteroid injections. Even though nobody gave Andrea any bad advice, she did not get any better. Finally she was referred to a shoulder expert.

After a thorough diagnostic workup this doctor found that Andrea suffered from a torn shoulder cuff and also had a large bony spur digging into one of the bursae that cushion the shoulder. Within months Andrea was scheduled for surgery. Her shoulder needed no new parts. The surgeon simply repaired the rotator cuff.

After the surgery Andrea's pain substantially subsided, but it took months of physical therapy to regain some mobility, and even longer to again take up the violin. Now, nine months after her operation, Andrea plays again—even professionally.

"I play comfortably for thirty minutes now," Andrea told her doctor during her last visit. "After sixty minutes I have to use ice, but I'll get there—thanks to you and my wonderful physical therapist."

Musicians are like athletes except that nonfunctioning joints are even worse for them. They have no down time. They repeat the same motion for hours on end. Most musicians have no concept of time. Like the ballerina with the red ballet slippers in Hans Christian Andersen's fairy tale, they just keep going on.

ROCHELLE F.

When she was forty years old, Rochelle's hip hurt. "I immediately assumed that it was osteoarthritis," she remembered twenty years later, "because everybody in my family—my mother, uncles and aunts—suffered from that disease."

Rochelle's answer to her arthritis was yoga. She stretched, bent, and twisted herself—and felt better.

"My pain increased whenever I did not exercise," Rochelle recalled, "so I kept up my yoga."

The arthritis did not stop Rochelle from going back to school. She went to Library School at Columbia University. After helping Ralph put their three children through college, Rochelle went to Bridgeport University and earned a master's degree in social work.

Rochelle's hip behaved, but in her fifties the joints of her fingers became extremely painful. The memory of her mother's crippled hands haunted her. Since she had been a librarian, books were Rochelle's first resort. She read a lot of books, but found occupational therapy journals most helpful.

"I bought a rubber reflexology ball and exercised my hands. I flexed and extended my fingers, and it helped my hands. I can do most things, though my hands tire easily. When I write for a long time, my hands cramp.

"I hate taking medication and avoid anti-inflammatory drugs like aspirin most of the time. I find that exercise and massages help. When I can afford it, I have a massage once a week."

Rochelle also became very interested in relaxation, meditation, and other methods of stress reduction. She uses these techniques successfully for her patients at one of Connecticut's most exclusive psychiatric care facilities.

"My X rays show that there is osteoarthritis in my hips, my knees, my back, and my hands. My head fights it," she asserts.

◆ ◆ ◆ ◆ ◆ ◆ ◆

Claude, Naomi, Rochelle, and Bernice have osteoarthritis. Andrea's shoulder joint was disabled by overuse. The initial treatment for all was the same: pain relief with anti-inflammatory medication and alternative methods, rest, ice when the joint was hurting acutely, heat to relieve the pain, and EXERCISE. Though three of the five patients eventually had surgery, this is usually not necessary. As they discovered almost immediately, osteoarthritis is an unglamorous, common disease that did not entitle them to much sympathy from family and friends.

Each of the five mourned the loss of the effortless way in which their body used to move. Naomi used to scamper over rocks as if she were a mountain goat. Claude skied for hours. Bernice embroidered and made her own clothes. Andrea never thought about how long she practiced her violin. Rochelle was the star of her yoga class.

All five worried about the impact of arthritis on their bodies and lifestyle. Would they limp? Be always in pain? Could they still work, travel, hike, go to art galleries, shop for clothes?

They knew, however, that they were lucky, because so much can be done for arthritis victims today. There are better drugs to manage pain, and judiciously prescribed exercise can maintain and protect joints.

Interestingly, the improved understanding of the role of exercise in the management of osteoarthritis is an outgrowth of momentous surgical strides in joint reconstruction. During the 1960s and 1970s Dr. John Charnley, a British surgeon, developed an artificial hip, which could replace a diseased one if necessary. The success with the hip stimulated interest in perfecting a workable total knee replacement. Today the function of most diseased joints can be improved surgically.

Surgery, however, is a last resort and should never be undertaken lightly. Most degenerative joint diseases are managed non-operatively.

◆ ◆ ◆ ◆ ◆ ◆ ◆

Let us now follow Naomi's medical history. Her family physician sent her to a rheumatologist (arthritis specialist), who confirmed the diagnosis, gave her a prescription, and sent her to a physical therapist. He also advised her to swim regularly and not to gain weight.

This regimen worked for a long time, but in the course of ten years, the hip continued to deteriorate. At first it hurt only when Naomi overdid things—stood too long or walked too much. Gradually it began to interfere with everyday activities. She hated to stand—on a bus, in the subway, in line at the theater or grocery store. At cocktail parties she parked herself on a chair. Going to museums and sight-seeing became difficult.

As the years passed, the pain was no longer localized in the hip. Naomi's whole body hurt so much that she wondered whether she did not have one of the systemic (affecting the whole body) forms of the disease. Her annual X rays showed continued deterioration; the hip also became less and less functional. A normal hip rotates 45° to each side. Each year Naomi's hip rotated a little less.

Naomi, stoic by nature, did not let pain interfere with her activities. She dragged her poor hip to work, to the supermarket, on the subway, on all-day hikes, even to Rome and Paris. After some of these bravura feats, her hip hurt so much that she went to bed as soon as she got home, even foregoing supper. When she hurt she was cranky and unpleasant to live with.

She popped aspirins and the closely related newer anti-arthritis medications. They helped, but eventually her stomach revolted.

She listened to her physician and physical therapist and exercised. She faithfully did her prescribed floor exercises and whenever possible went to the pool two to three times a week. This regimen maintained the tone of the muscles that surround her hip. She loved the swimming. In the water she felt like her former athletic self.

For many years Naomi's hip only hurt during the day, but eventually the pain continued even after she crept under her electric blanket. Was it time to have a new hip?

Even though Naomi's doctor offered support and professional advice, he made it clear that he wanted her to decide if and when she should have a new hip. "Remember," he said, "there can be complications—infections, loosening—and nobody knows yet how long an artificial hip lasts. Ten, fifteen years perhaps, and you are still young. If we operate now, you may outlive your artificial joint and need a revision (repair job)."

Eventually Naomi's pain became so bad that she chose the surgery. She hoped that a new, pain-free left hip might protect her right hip, which was showing mild deterioration.

The years of swimming and floor exercises paid off. Naomi recovered very quickly. A few days after the operation she walked on two crutches to give the new hip a chance to heal, then one crutch, then a cane. After six weeks she walked unaided. After three months she took a ten-mile hike. Her entire body was pain-free.

Naomi, however, was not through with osteoarthritis. The disease is now affecting her right knee, left hip, right shoulder, right elbow, and lower back. The knee is by far the worst. When it was last x-rayed, most of the cartilage that protects the end of the bones, allowing for pain-free movement, was gone.

Sometimes Naomi "hurts all over." Sometimes she has back pain; sometimes the knee is very bad. Most of the time Naomi feels pretty good. She trusts her doctors, and like Bernice, Claude, Andrea, and Rochelle, she has learned to live with her disease.

By now Naomi knows her body very well. She knows which movements will relieve pain, when to rest, when to take a painkiller, what shoes to wear, and what not to do.

She also knows an awful lot about arthritis, and that helps. When she goes to see a new doctor or therapist (medical care is so specialized today that you are likely to deal with many different professionals) she understands what they are talking about. Her understanding helps her participate in making decisions about her treatment, to do her exercises properly, to ask relevant questions. Her knowledge keeps fear at bay.

Claude, Bernice, Andrea, and Rochelle are also doing well. Each has a slightly different attitude on how to manage his or her disease. All have serious joint problems; none are invalids. Throughout this book we will meet many other patients who also have come to terms with their disease.

Since you are reading this book, you—or a member of your family—may suffer from osteoarthritis, and you have to learn to deal with it. When asked how to live for a long time, William Osler, one of the world's greatest physicians, said, "Get a chronic disease and take good care of it."

Osler was right. Patients who participate in their own care and understand their own disease fare much better than those who either ignore their pain or totally abdicate responsibility for their own health. It is extremely important to select health care providers (the term here applies to all the many specialists involved in your medical care) who are both competent and compassionate—those who are willing to spend some time with you.

Medical care is undergoing tremendous changes, and doctors, once firmly enthroned on a pedestal, are now considered fallible. Today, doctors take a patient's wishes into account, especially when the decisions involve a chronic, non-life-threatening disease like arthritis, for which there is no standard treatment or cure. No doctor, for instance, will insist that you undergo surgery. Claude's and Naomi's doctors told them that they would actually make the decision as to whether they wanted new joints or not. Doctors also will not insist that you take a specific drug.

Even though doctors want your input, they often are not very skilled at talking with patients. A recent health care survey reported in the *Wall Street Journal* found that doctors usually interrupt patients within the first eighteen seconds of an interview and then spend less than two minutes of a twenty-minute session sharing information.

Doctors often insist on speaking a language of their own. You may not understand what they are saying when they talk of ulnar drifts, marginal changes in the trapeziometacarpal joint, disk space narrowing, or osteophyte spur formation—or tell you that you can take your medication "ad lib." You may have to educate your doctor by insisting that he or she spend adequate time talking to you in plain English.

You will also get more out of your visit if you have done your homework. It is helpful not to waste precious time asking about simple facts that you could have easily learned on your own. It is wise to study and come prepared with a list of meaningful questions.

You are now ready to continue learning about osteoarthritis, the joints it affects, the drugs and the exercises, the surgical options, and the many other aspects of living with a chronic disease. Do not "tough out" joint pain on your own. According to the Arthritis Foundation, you should see a doctor when the following warning signs occur:

- Persistent pain and stiffness on arising
- Pain and tenderness or swelling in one or more joints
- Recurrence of these symptoms, especially when they involve more than one joint
- Recurrent or persistent pain and stiffness in the neck, lower back, knees, and other joints

◆ CHAPTER ◆

2

First Things First: The Medical Treatment of Osteoarthritis

Every person's body hurts some of the time. Usually the aches and pains disappear on their own after a few days. When pain persists, we go to see a doctor. Usually we first consult a general practitioner, general internist, or orthopedist. We may also consult, or be referred to, a rheumatologist, who specializes in arthritis care.

There are many kinds of arthritis (See Chapter 3 and Appendix I), and part of your initial evaluation consists of determining whether you indeed have arthritis. Additional evaluations will determine what kind of arthritis you suffer from.

Your Doctor, Your Partner

The first visit to a new doctor, especially one who deals with chronic diseases, is important. It is the beginning of a partnership. You will have to decide whether you like and trust this doctor. Does he or she seem competent and kind? Listen to you? Show respect? Does the doctor explain matters in "plain English," or does he or she insist on using medical jargon that you don't fully understand? Will the physician be aware that medical care is expensive and help you use your financial resources wisely? Will he or she perceive you as a human being and not only an assemblage of pain, bones, and joints?

The doctor, too, is entitled to evaluate new patients. Will they be truthful? Trust the doctor? Show respect? Will they make a sincere attempt to follow the prescribed treatment to the best of their ability?

Initial Visit

You will make your doctor's job easier, and derive more benefit from your initial visit, if you are well prepared. It is helpful if you bring any medical records, X rays, or blood test data that you have. It will save time, and ensure good results, if you write down your questions, your symptoms, other diseases you are suffering from, and accurate information on all the *medications* that you are taking (see Preparation for Initial Visit, page 16).

The initial visit focus will be accurately diagnosing your disease. The first and most important task is to determine whether the pain stems from arthritis or whether it is the symptom of another disease. If the doctor determines that you have arthritis, he or she must then identify the type of arthritis you have.

To answer these questions the doctor will

- take a medical history
- examine you from head to toe
- order and evaluate the necessary diagnostic tests

Here is what this short list means.

Medical History

Symptoms Related to the Present Complaint

The most crucial questions relate to a detailed description of your symptoms. For musculoskeletal diseases this will indicate whether you suffer from arthritis or whether the joint pain is due to an injury of soft tissues such as ligaments, tendons, or bursae. Think about some of the following questions commonly asked during the initial visit to an arthritis specialist:

Onset of Pain: Did it start suddenly? Did it start gradually over the course of months?

Type of Pain: How long does it last? How intense is it? When does it occur? At night? In the evening? During the day? When you exercise? After you exercise? When you are resting?

Mobility: Do you feel stiff? In the morning? After sitting for a long time? Can you walk easily on flat ground? Can you climb stairs? Can you get up easily from the floor? From the bed? From an armless chair? From the toilet? Can you easily get out of a car? A bathtub?

Lifestyle: Are your symptoms interfering with things you want or need to do? Do you have trouble with recreational activities? Sports? Do you have trouble dressing, brushing your hair, eating, doing your work, opening doors, opening cans, buttoning clothes, tying shoelaces, turning faucets? Do you have trouble walking?

It is important for the physician to be aware of all your other medical problems (such as heart disease, high blood pressure, diabetes, and kidney disease), as well as of all the medications (prescription and over-the-counter) that you may be taking.

Physical Examination

In addition to a routine examination (taking of blood pressure, listening to the heart and lungs) the doctor will examine your joints and see how they function while you walk, bend, and stretch. Hands and feet are carefully examined. The doctor will also evaluate the strength and stability of your joints and the grip strength of your hands.

X Rays

By now a skilled examiner will probably have a good idea of whether and where you have arthritis, and may confirm the diagnosis by ordering X rays. These will also give an indication of the severity of the arthritis. Interestingly, there is not always a correlation between the extent of the osteoarthritis as it appears on the X ray and the degree of pain and dysfunction.

Osteoarthritis does not appear overnight, although acute pain may seem to you to occur suddenly. Most joints deteriorate over months, even years. You may have only a little discomfort, which most people tend to ignore or discount, until the disease reaches a certain threshold. Then the joint suddenly becomes very painful. With some luck, a well thought-out medical program will make the joint functional again

Preparation for Initial Visit

SYMPTOMS Be able to describe your symptoms as accurately as you can, including what you can and cannot do. Do you have pain during the day, during exercise, after exercise, at night? Note the progression of your symptoms. When did you note the first symptoms? Did they start suddenly or slowly? Information like this helps determine whether the pain is truly associated with a joint or whether it is the result of an injury to some soft tissue such as a ligament, a tendon, or a bursa.

MEDICATION Make a list of all the medications you take, both prescription and over-the-counter. Include those you take only once in a while (sleeping pills) or seasonally (allergy pills). If the physician prescribes a new drug, ask

- whether the medication is for pain only
- how long you will be taking it
- whether it can be taken together with aspirin or Tylenol
- whether it has any side effects, and what these may be
- whether it interacts with other medication you take and if so, how to schedule the various medications
- what to do when you forget to take a particular dosage

EXERCISE, REST, DIET Explain your lifestyle, including exercises you do, rests you take, and diets you are on or have tried in the past. Report activities you would like to do and cannot.

QUESTIONS Do not be afraid to discuss your fears and anxieties. If indicated, voice complaints about your treatment. Adjustments can usually be made that may make you—and your doctor—happier.

and reduce your pain. Sometimes joints function well in spite of extensive damage. The reverse can be true: seemingly minor deterioration may cause major pain and dysfunction.

WHO TREATS ARTHRITIS?

Arthritis care is best delivered by a team of health professionals. These include

Internists, family practitioners, rheumatologists, who

- mastermind your overall care, prescribe drugs, and refer you to other members of the arthritis team

Physical therapists, who

- observe how you use your body
- teach you exercises that will keep your joints as functional as possible and strengthen the muscles surrounding the affected joint
- help you develop an overall exercise program

Occupational therapists, who

- help you use your joints in the most efficient, least painful manner
- make splints that protect painful joints
- provide you with gadgets that make common tasks easier

Dietitians, who

- help you to develop a sound eating plan

Nurse practitioners, who

- assist the physician in supervising your care and may adjust your medication, rest and exercise schedule

Orthopedic surgeons, who

- perform surgery including arthroscopy or joint replacement. Orthopedic surgeons are often the first physicians consulted by patients suffering from severe muscle or joint pain. They may also provide second opinions as to whether or when surgery is indicated.

Social workers, who

- are trained to help you sort out the many emotional and financial problems associated with having a chronic disease

Physiatrists (rehabilitation specialists), who

- help patients with chronic pain and other problems not addressed by other treatment modalities

Together these health professionals will teach you to

- control your pain with drugs or by other methods
- take care of your joints through a combination of rest and exercise
- reduce stress on your joints by maintaining an acceptable body weight
- maintain a reasonable lifestyle

They also help you decide if and when to have surgery.

Subsequent chapters of this book, written by health professionals specializing in arthritis care at Columbia Presbyterian Medical Center, detail various aspects of treatment. This chapter presents a general game plan appropriate for most patients.

Self-Care

Osteoarthritis is a disease that requires informed self-care. Your primary care physician will prescribe drugs, teach you how to manage your disease, and explain how to do exercises properly. But arthritis is a chronic, unpredictable disease, and you are the captain of your health care team. The fact that you are reading this book is an indication that you understand your responsibility to yourself.

Before talking about treatment, let me urge you to maintain a positive outlook about triumphing over your arthritis. Developing a healthy attitude toward chronic disease is more than half the battle.

Many people believe that arthritis is synonymous with old age. You may therefore be reluctant to acknowledge to yourself that you suffer from osteoarthritis. But it is not true that osteoarthritis and old age are one and the same.

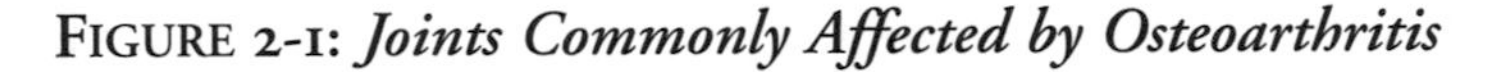

FIGURE 2-1: *Joints Commonly Affected by Osteoarthritis*

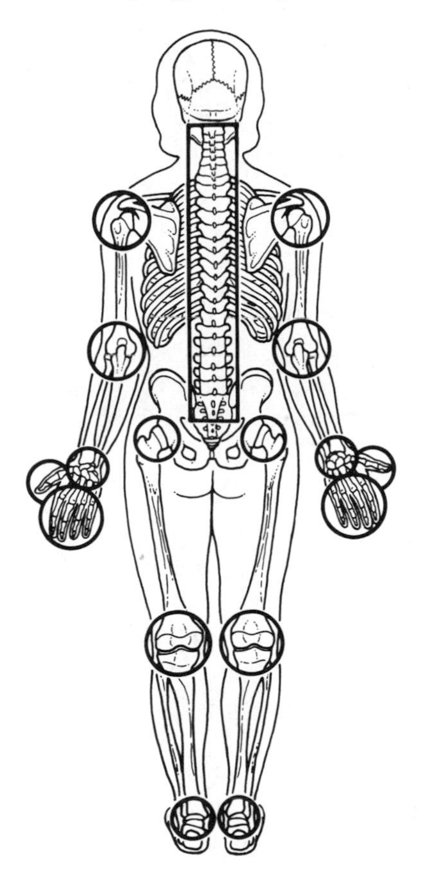

The following joints are commonly affected by osteoarthritis. These joints are usually hardworking and weight-bearing. Most can now be reconstructed surgically. The next chapter provides additional details about the structure of specific joints.

Arthritis, like all other diseases, takes its toll. You may have to give up certain activities and modify others. You may have to devote some time to doing exercises. You have to deal with pain. *But* you do not have to "give up," feel debility is inevitable, or that your condition cannot be improved.

Osteoarthritis is better than many other disorders. It does not affect your mental capacities. Total joint replacement offers a permanent cure for some major joints. A better understanding of body mechanics, the role of exercise, improved drug therapy, laborsaving devices, and adaptive lifestyle modifications will enable you to lead an enjoyable existence.

During your initial visits to the doctor, you and your physician will develop a plan that enables you to function in spite of your arthritis. Even though such plans are highly individualized and require frequent adjustment, the broad outline given here applies to most patients.

Treatment Plan

It would be nice if, once diagnosed, osteoarthritis could be treated by a simple medication. Except for joint replacement surgery, which is reviewed at length in the second part of this book, there is as yet no definite treatment that reverses osteoarthritis.

Drug Therapy

Most patients expect to leave the doctor's office with a prescription for a new drug. Indeed, arthritis victims are a boon to the drug industry. Certain medications are essential for those suffering from the inflammatory forms of the disease. For the patient suffering from osteoarthritis, drugs have only one principal and crucial function: alleviating pain.

The choice of drugs to accomplish this relief is very important and is discussed at length in Chapter 4 and in Appendix III. Most of the drugs used are relatives of aspirin. Because they are not steroids (like cortisone), this family of drugs goes by the name of nonsteroidal anti-inflammatory drugs, or NSAIDs.

It cannot be stressed often enough, however, that no drug will cure your arthritis. Aspirin and many of the newer nonsteroidal anti-inflammatory drugs (NSAIDs) frequently have unpleasant side effects. You may thus be better off alleviating your pain with acetaminophen or even propoxyphene hydrochloride (Darvon). Continual, clear communication with your doctor will assure that you'll receive the most helpful medication.

Exercise

There are two types of exercise for patients suffering from osteoarthritis: *therapeutic* and *aerobic*. Therapeutic exercises preserve mobility and strengthen the muscles surrounding the affected joint. These exercises are discussed in Chapter 5 and, as appropriate, in Part II of this book. As everybody with chronic back disease knows, therapeutic exercises can relieve or lessen the pain associated with musculoskeletal disorders.

Establish a routine for when to do your exercises: before breakfast, at bedtime, or while watching a favorite soap opera or news commentator.

Aerobic exercises that maintain cardiovascular health and improve overall physical fitness are important for everyone, including people with arthritis. A regular exercise program improves muscle tone, burns off calories, and prevents depression.

It is of course most gratifying for patients to continue with the sport they took part in before they developed osteoarthritis. Often patients may have to modify or tone down the activity: racewalking instead of running, doubles tennis matches instead of singles, golf instead of handball. Patients with more advanced arthritis may be better off with low impact (nonjoint stressing) exercises like swimming, walking, or use of stationary bicycles, rowing machines, or track machines.

Rest and Joint Protection

Regularly scheduled rest periods that promote relaxation and ready muscles for the next round of exercise or activity are a crucial aspect of the overall treatment plan.

Affected joints should be protected as much as possible. Canes take pressure from the body weight off the hips and knees. A splint, worn at night, protects wrists and finger joints. A soft neck collar or a cervical pillow protects the cervical spine. Labor-saving kitchen equipment reduces stress on the finger joints. A carefully adjusted chair reduces back strain. Chapter 6 discusses such measures in greater detail.

Pain Relief Techniques

Pain is what brought you to the doctor in the first place. Lessening this pain as much as possible is a chief goal of therapy. Pain can often be relieved temporarily without drugs through the application of heat or cold. Learning to use your joints properly is another approach. Chapter 6 reviews commonly used techniques.

OVERALL TREATMENT PLAN

DIAGNOSIS	During the initial visit the doctor takes a thorough medical history, performs a physical examination, and orders an X ray of the affected joints. This will enable him or her to confirm or rule out whether or not you suffer from osteoarthritis.
DRUG THERAPY	The overwhelming purpose of drug therapy for patients suffering from OA is to relieve pain. Medications used for this purpose include aspirin, Tylenol, any of the newer nonsteroidal anti-inflammatory drugs (NSAIDs) discussed in Chapter 4 and in Appendix III, and miscellaneous other agents. Therapeutic response to these analgesic drugs is highly individualized, and you may have to try several drugs to find the one that suits you best.
EXERCISE	A regular exercise is essential. Chapter 5 reviews suitable exercises for patients suffering from osteoarthritis.
DIET	Weight loss or weight maintenance is part of the plan. Excess body weight stresses the weight-bearing joints often affected by OA. Moreover, joint pain promotes a sedentary lifestyle. It is

Weight Control

You know even without consulting a physician that excess body weight puts additional stress on the weight-bearing joints. Overweight also impairs overall function and causes stress to the circulatory system. For more details, see Chapter 7.

	therefore important for patients to be aware of their body weight.
REST	Frequent rest periods and protection of the affected joint through the use of splints, canes, or walkers prevents additional damage to affected joints.
PAIN RELIEF TECHNIQUES	Relief of pain by the local application of heat or or cold, paraffin baths, and other means improves joint mobility.
REDUCING JOINT STRESS	Reducing stress on joints during routine activities by rearranging home, office, and car, as appropriate. Maintaining good posture while lying in bed, sitting, and standing.
SURGERY	Patients suffering from OA are the principal beneficiaries of the joint replacement techniques developed during the past twenty years. Having major surgery is nevertheless an important decision to be made jointly by the patient and his or her physician. Chapter 8 discusses factors to be considered during the decision-making process. Specific techniques used to relieve OA of the hip, knee, back, shoulder, hand, and foot are reviewed in Part II of this book.

Surgery

One of the most important tasks of the rheumatologist or internist is to help you decide whether or when to have surgery. Important factors are the extent of the disease, the intensity of the pain, and how much these factors interfere with your life. A patient's age, work, and lifestyle are also considered. An elderly man may be perfectly happy to give up hiking and walk with a cane. A ballet dancer may not. Such considerations are discussed in Chapter 8.

Once the diagnosis is established and initial treatment prescribed, most physicians ask new patients to report back four weeks later unless the condition requires more immediate follow-up. At the second visit it is possible to determine whether the drugs and exercises have helped and whether the acute pain has subsided. Prepare for this follow-up visit as you did for the initial one.

Preparation for Follow-up Visit

The purpose of this visit is to evaluate the initial treatment plan and modify it as necessary.

BE HONEST. Doctors know that most of their patients neglect some aspects of their treatment. It is, however, important that you report accurately on what you did or did not do.

Again, prepare a checklist reminding you of the topics you wish to discuss with the doctor.

- **Pain:** Is it better, worse, or the same as before?
- **Drugs:** Did they help decrease your pain? Did you take the full dose? Did you take additional pills?
- **Exercise:** Did you do your exercises? Did they help? Did you see a physical therapist? Join an exercise class? Bring in your exercise diary if you kept one.
- **Mood:** How has your mood been? Did you sleep well? How was your appetite?
- **Food:** Did you cut out some fattening foods? If applicable, bring your food diary.

◆ CHAPTER ◆

3

Osteoarthritis and the Joints of the Body

What Is Arthritis?

The word *arthritis* comes from the Greek words *arthro* (joint) and *itis,* an ending always meaning inflammation. Arthritis simply means "joint inflammation." Most forms of the disease are characterized by painful, swollen joints. The cause of this inflammation, however, differs from one form of arthritis to another. Osteoarthritis, also called degenerative joint disease, is by far the most common form of arthritis.

Osteoarthritis affects 121 persons out of 1,000 between the ages of eighteen and seventy-nine; rheumatoid arthritis, the next most common form of arthritis, affects only 9 out of 1,000 people. While the various forms of arthritis can affect people of all ages, the prevalence of osteoarthritis increases dramatically with age.

A Disease by Any Other Name

Knowing that arthritis is a family name does not end the confusion about what to call this group of disorders. They also go by the following names:

rheumatic diseases

connective tissue diseases

collagen diseases

musculoskeletal disorders

The word *rheumatism,* like *arthritis,* is historic. *Rheuma* comes from the Greek and means "a watery discharge" and refers to the fact that joints affected by arthritis often are swollen. Moreover, the disease seemed associated with cold, wet weather. Today the term *rheumatic diseases* is synonymous with arthritis. Doctors treating arthritis are called rheumatologists.

Connective tissue, like arthritis and rheumatism, is a general term referring to the material that holds the various structures of the body together. Examples of connective tissue are bone, cartilage, skin, arteries, tendons, and ligaments. Other examples are the thin membranes enclosing each cell and tissues that hold groups of cells together to form organs. Diseases that involve these connective tissues are referred to as *connective tissue diseases.*

Collagen, a protein, is a principal constituent of connective tissue. In some forms of arthritis (rheumatoid arthritis, systemic lupus erythematosus, scleroderma) the body is believed to attack its own collagen-containing joint cartilage. These autoimmune diseases are commonly referred to as *collagen diseases.*

Finally, since any disease involving the joints also affects the muscles, doctors often talk of *musculoskeletal diseases.*

Major Forms of Arthritis

The hallmarks of the major forms of arthritis are listed in Table 3-1.

The Parts of the Whole

Since osteoarthritis affects the joints of the body, let us look at these structures and their components in greater detail. A joint, the meeting place of two or more bones, is so complex that it is often thought of as an organ. Joints come in many shapes and sizes, each perfectly adapted to its specific function. Figure 3-5 shows the schematized shape of various joints. Part II of this book provides additional

TABLE 3-1: *Major Forms of Arthritis*

Disease	Description	Most Common In
Ankylosing spondylitis	Form of arthritis affecting the spine. Treatment includes anti-inflammatory drugs and exercise.	Young men
Gout	Long associated with gluttony, gout is actually a metabolic disorder. The disease is now successfully treated with drugs.	Middle-aged men
Lyme arthritis	So-called because the first cases of this novel disease were discovered twenty years ago in the town of Lyme, Connecticut. Lyme arthritis is caused by *Borrelia burgdorferi,* an infectious disease agent transmitted by a deer tick. The initial bite often forms a big red spot about two inches in diameter. After a number of days or weeks patients may develop an array of symptoms including a type of arthritis that waxes and wanes and migrates from joint to joint. The disease usually responds to a timely injection of antibiotics.	
Osteoarthritis (OA)	Characterized by the degeneration of the cartilage that covers the ends of the bone. The disease attacks *only* isolated joints and does not involve the internal organs. Treatment: subject of this book.	Most common form of arthritis; incidence increases dramatically with age.
Rheumatoid arthritis (RA)	RA is a chronic, autoimmune disease characterized by a self-perpetuating inflammation of the thin layer of tissue lining the joint capsule (synovial membrane). RA and OA are often confused. RA is, however, a very different, much more severe systemic disease (involving the entire body). Patients often are tired, lose weight, and suffer from anemia. RA commonly affects symmetric joints (both knees, thumbs, elbows, hips, etc.). The disease varies in severity. Because both diseases cause joint pain and swelling, some of the same drugs are used for their treatment. (See Chapter 4.)	Most prevalent form of inflamatory arthritis; most commonly affects young women.
Systemic lupus erythematosus	Another autoimmune collagen disease, often affecting the internal organs, especially the kidneys and even the brain. Treatment: various drugs, antimalarials, corticosteroids.	Most common in women of childbearing age.

For other rheumatic diseases see Appendix I.

information about specific joints commonly affected by OA. This chapter examines the individual building blocks of all joints, consisting of

- *bone* covered by a layer of
- *articular cartilage*, which in turn consists of
    - *collagen*
    - *proteoglycans*
    - *water*

Bones

The body's solid framework is composed of extremely strong, hollow cylinders of bone. The ends of these cylinders are flared to provide the largest surface for joint contact.

The skeleton consists of approximately three hundred bones that provide the body with its solid framework and protect the delicate inner organs. The individual bones are connected by 143 joints.

At one time it was thought that, once formed, structural tissues like bone or cartilage were relatively inert. Today we know that even seemingly inert tissues are constantly turned over. Remodeling and repair of bone is carried out by two special types of cells. The *osteoclasts* remove bone and the *osteoblasts* form new bone. Both types of cells participate in the mending of broken bones.

The bulk of bone is extremely rigid. The joint edge of the bone, however, consists of a thin layer of *subchondral bone,* which is slightly more elastic than the bone itself, thereby acting as a shock absorber.

The overall structure of a long bone is shown in Figure 3-1. As you can see, bone does not have a solid, uniform structure.

Articular Cartilage

Articular hyaline cartilage is the translucent, gristlelike, shock-absorbing tissue covering the ends of the bones. Anyone who has ever examined the gristle that connects a chicken drumstick with its thighbone knows what articular cartilage looks like.

Articular cartilage is a very remarkable tissue. When healthy it is more slippery than ice, permitting the joint surfaces to glide over one

FIGURE 3-1: *Schematic View of a Long Bone*

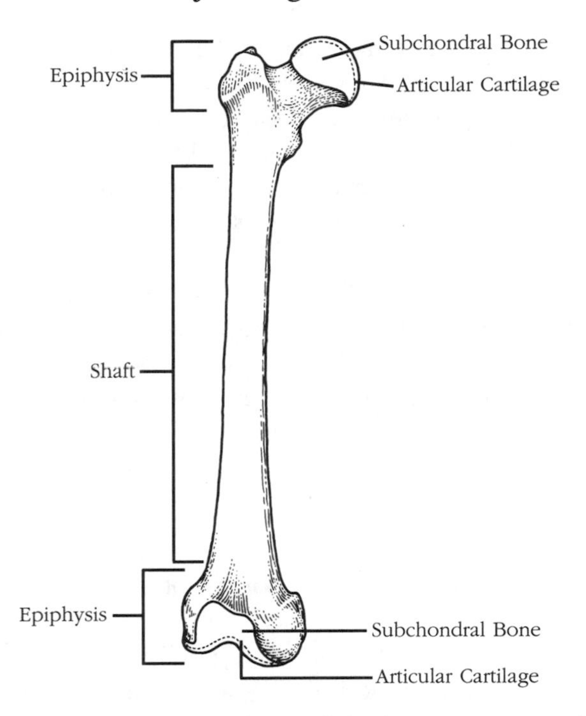

The Shaft: The shaft is the central portion of the bone, consisting of relatively unbending, dense connective tissue providing rigidity.
The Epiphysis: Growth, during the first fifteen to twenty years of life, takes place in the epiphyses, the ends of the bone.
Subchondral Bone: Directly under the cartilage is a layer of subchondral ("under cartilage") bone that is more porous and is replaced more frequently by new bone than the more highly calcified bone of the shaft. Upon impact subchondral bone can absorb some of the stress. Subchondral bone becomes less metabolically active with age, a fact that might contribute to the osteoarthritic process.
Articular Cartilage: The arrangement of the collagen and proteoglycan fibrils within the cartilage is such that they distribute the stress created by movement. The stress is highest in the weight-bearing joints, such as the hips and knees, but can be considerable in other, smaller joints.

another effortlessly during an entire lifetime. Cartilage is actually a network consisting mostly of intertwined strands of *collagen* and *proteoglycans.* These solid constituents, however, account for only 20 percent of the cartilage. Some 65 to 80 percent of the articular cartilage is fluid, mostly water.

Collagen

Collagen is the body's most widely distributed family of proteins. Eighteen different species of these fibrous proteins have been identified so far. Depending on their ultimate function, the collagen fibers may be transparent (cornea); ropelike (tendons); weight-bearing (bone); adapted to be woven into sheets (skin); or endowed with shock-absorbing elasticity, tensile strength, and stiffness (articular cartilage).

Like other proteins, collagen consists of chains of linked amino acids. These amino acid chains are grouped together to form polypeptides. In collagen, three distinct strands of polypeptides wind around one another in a helical fashion. Figure 3-2 shows a schematic representation of various types of collagen.

Proteoglycans

The other major structural constituents of articular cartilage are the proteoglycans—another biochemical building material that is a combination of protein and sugars. Like proteins, the proteoglycans are assembled from smaller subunits. When magnified under an electron microscope, the proteoglycans look like spherical dishbrushes. In articular cartilage strands of proteoglycans units attached to a "backbone" intertwine with the collagen fibers to form a dense mesh. Proteoglycans provide cartilage with resiliency, enabling it to stretch and then reassume its original shape.

Cartilage Turnover

Cartilage, like bone, is constantly "turned over." Special cartilage-forming cells called *chrondrocytes* are dispersed throughout the cartilage to manufacture collagens and proteoglycans.

The chondrocytes can also release enzymes that destroy both collagen and proteoglycans. The chondrocytes are responsible for the synthesis and development of the cartilage, its maintenance, and apparently even its degradation in osteoarthritis. Both the formation of new cartilage and its degradation by enzymes are believed to play a major role in the disease.

FIGURE 3-2: *Arrangement of Collagen Fibers in Various Tissues (Schematic View)*

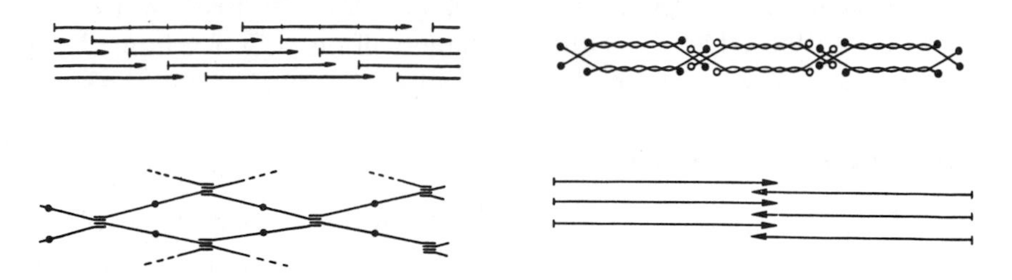

The type and arrangement of the collagen fibers determine the nature of the specific connective tissue. *Reproduced by permission of Sergio A. Jiminez, M.D., adapted from Martin et al. in* Trends in Biochemical Science *(1985).*

Architecture of Articular Cartilage

Nature never leaves anything to chance. Even something as thin as articular cartilage is carefully structured so that it provides the joint with mechanical strength.

So far scientists have noted that the cartilage is arranged into four layers, which differ from one another with respect to

- the nature of the collagen fibers
- the ratio between collagen and proteoglycans
- the distribution of the chrondrocytes throughout the articular cartilage

Here is how the individual layers of cartilage are structured:

1. The outermost (surface) layer of cartilage is thin and consists mostly of fine collagen fibrils.
2. The next layer (10–20 percent of total thickness) consists of chondrocytes and collagen fibrils arranged parallel to the joint surface.

3. The middle layer (30 percent of total thickness) has broad collagen fibrils and the highest proteoglycan content.
4. The deepest layer (30 percent of total thickness), closest to the bone surface, has the largest collagen fibrils, often arranged perpendicular to the bone surface.

Fluid Content of Cartilage

Like other tissues, cartilage is mostly water. Water plays a major role in providing cartilage with its shock-absorbing properties. During mechanical impact, fluid exudes from cartilage, to be reabsorbed during relaxation. In this way cartilage acts like a wet sponge that releases water and cushions blows when compressed.

Structure of a Synovial Joint

Most of the joints considered in this book are synovial joints. This means that they are enclosed in a

- *joint capsule*, lined with a
- *synovial membrane,* which produces the
- *synovial fluid,* which lubricates the joint.

Even the most perfectly designed joint, however, could not perform its function without

- *muscles, ligaments, and tendons.* The latter are often cushioned by small, liquid-filled pouches, the
- *bursae.*

Let us now examine these joint components in greater detail.

Joint Capsule

The mobile synovial joints, like the hip and knee, are surrounded by a capsule consisting of two layers. A tough, fibrous outer layer holds the bones of the joint together and prevents the joint from overextending. An inner lining, the thin synovium, produces the synovial fluid that lubricates and nourishes the cartilage. Both layers of the joint capsule are amply supplied with blood and lymph and equipped with pain-sensing nerve endings. The synovial membrane is in large part responsible for the pain and swelling characteristic of arthritis. When inflamed, it swells and thickens. Instead of the normally clear, viscous synovial fluid, the membrane secretes puslike material laden with white blood cells.

Joint Space

Healthy joints have a well-defined joint space permitting free movement. This space is filled with synovial fluid that helps lubricate the joint. During periods of inflammation, the volume of this fluid can increase dramatically, thus contributing to the swelling often seen in arthritic joints.

Muscles, Tendons, and Ligaments

The principal function of the musculoskeletal system is to enable the body to move at will. All joints are equipped with nerves that transmit messages. Ligaments, tendons, and muscles do the actual work. Arthritis does not affect the muscles that operate the joints.

However, because of arthritis pain, sufferers may avoid using the affected joint. This tendency often gradually leads to muscle deterioration. In turn, the loss of muscle tissue may alter the proper joint alignment, promoting disuse and deformity. This is why exercises that specifically maintain muscle strength are such an important aspect of treatment.

Bursae

In most joints the ligaments and tendons are cushioned by small, fluid-filled bursae. Stress, overuse, or injury may inflame such bursae, causing *bursitis.* A frozen shoulder is a very common form of bursitis.

Types of Joints

Given the number of different tasks the skeleton must perform, it is surprising that nature evolved only three types of joints: the synarthroidal joints, amphiarthroidal joints, and diarthroidal joints.

Synarthroidal Joints

Bones that usually stay put with respect to one another, like the plates that form the skull, are connected by synarthroidal joints. These joints are not affected by arthritis.

Amphiarthroidal Joints

Fibrocartilaginous material forms the amphiarthroidal joint, permitting some minor movement of the bones with respect to one another. The intervertebral discs of the spinal column are one example of amphiarthroidal joints.

Even though they cause humankind much grief because they wear, degenerate, and herniate, the intervertebral discs do not develop typical osteoarthritis.

Diarthroidal (Synovial) Joints

The highly mobile joints that play such an important part in arthritis are of the diarthroidal (or synovial) type. Even though these joints come in various shapes (hinge, ball and socket, saddle, gliding, pivot, and ellipsoidal), they all have the same basic structure. Figure 3-4 illustrates the overall structure of a synovial joint, and Figure 3-3 shows types of synovial joints found throughout the body.

OVERALL JOINT FUNCTION

Stress

Joints, especially those that bear weight, are highly stressed. Take the hip and knee joints, for example. Each time you take a step they experience a force three times your body weight. In the course of a single day, each joint is stressed hundreds of times. The body reduces the impact by flexing the joint and by distributing the load among the muscles that operate the joint, the cartilage, and even the underlying bone. With age and disease the cushioning effects decrease and people automatically learn to step more slowly and cautiously. Simple devices can decrease the load put onto a joint. Well-designed shoes with cushioned soles will help to reduce the impact loads that the joints experience.

FIGURE 3-3: *Examples of Synovial Joints*

HINGE

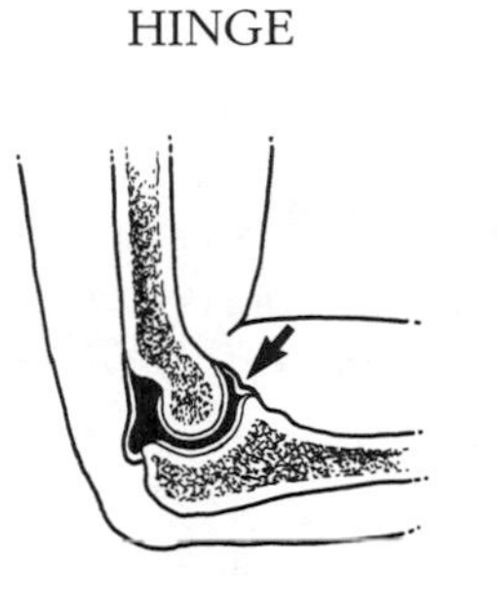

Elbow

BALL AND SOCKET

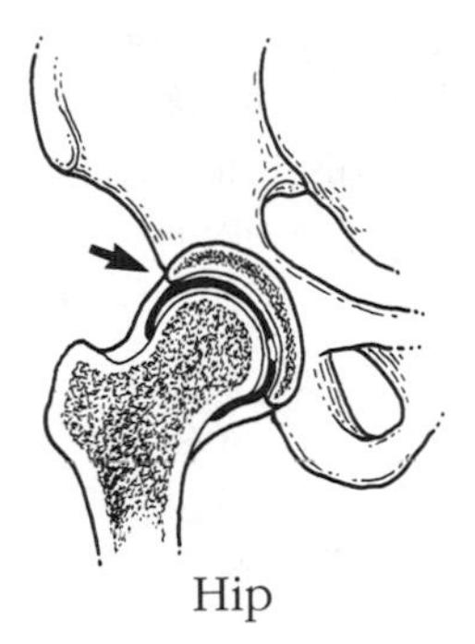

Hip

SADDLE

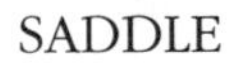

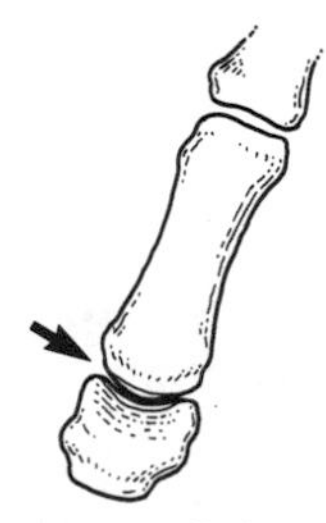

Base of thumb

GLIDING

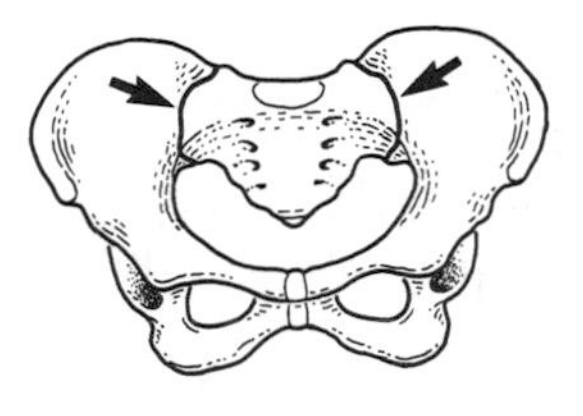

Sacroiliac

PIVOT

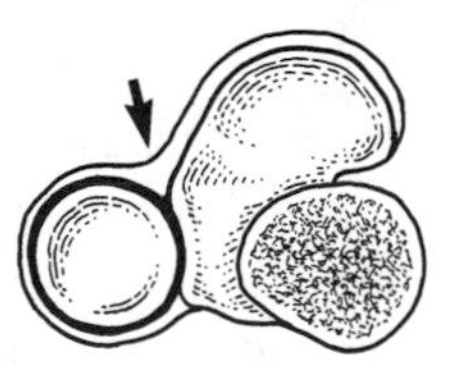

Radius-ulna

ELLIPSOIDAL

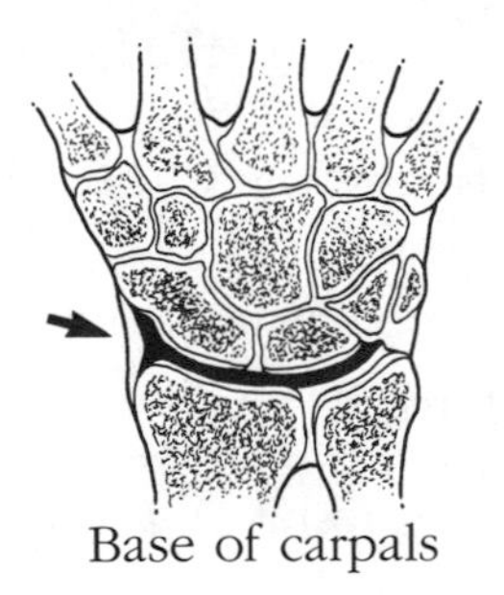

Base of carpals

Synovial joints have joint space between the bones they connect. This space insures the mobility of the joint. As illustrated, the shape and type of joint dictate its motion. Most of the joints you are familiar with are synovial joints.

A cane, for example, can absorb one third of body weight, sparing the knee and hip joints at every step.

Mobility

Throughout this book there will be much emphasis on joint mobility. Marked loss of mobility or reduced range of motion is the first clinical symptom of osteoarthritis. It is interesting to note, however, that loss of mobility begins in infancy. The joints of a baby are much more flexible than those of even a five-year-old child.

Joint surfaces in synovial joints are highly polished. These perfectly smooth surfaces minimize friction as the joint moves. In a healthy joint the "high gloss" is maintained by constant repair and renewal of the articular surface. Friction is further reduced by the presence of lubricating synovial fluid and by its flow pattern during compression of the joint.

Stability

It is as important for a joint to be stable as it is for it to be mobile. Stability is conferred by the shape of the joint (note that the surface of the bone within the joint is always slightly curved); the restraining forces of ligaments, muscles, and tendons; and, finally, by the viscous synovial fluid. Deterioration of any of these may lead to a highly unstable joint.

How Osteoarthritis Develops

There are many ways in which osteoarthritis begins. Abnormal stress on the cartilage is a major suspect. Scientists are investigating how these disease-initiating stresses differ from the constant, everyday compression, oscillation, twisting, and turning to which cartilage is subjected. Damage to other structures of the joint, such as the ligaments or tendons, may result in abnormal loading of the cartilage and lead to osteoarthritis.

Normally the body anticipates a forthcoming impact, such as that caused by each step during walking, and part of the action's force is

FIGURE 3-4: *Overall Structure of a Synovial Joint*

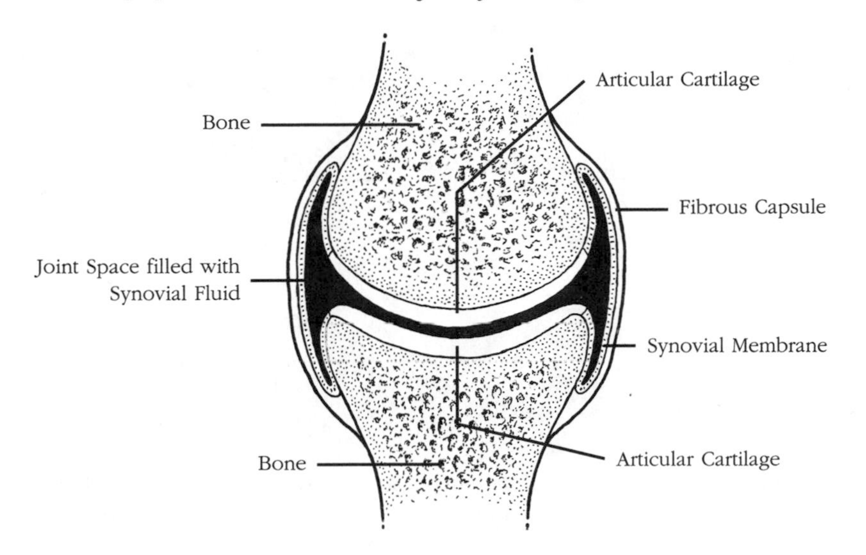

All synovial joints have the same basic structure.

absorbed by the preparedness of the supporting joint structure. However, a rapid, unexpected impact may cause small fractures in the underlying bone or injure the articular cartilage itself.

The chrondrocytes attempt an unsuccessful repair. There may be bone spur formation or bony overgrowth, both of which aggravate the condition, further impairing motion. Once initiated, the disease process is aggravated because articular cartilage cannot easily repair itself.

This trauma to the cartilage causes a disorganization of the collagen network and promotes water retention. These changes may initiate the disease process. The smooth cartilage surface may become pitted and frayed. Eventually the cartilage may lose some of its ability to hold fluid, thereby becoming less able to withstand loading. This irregular joint surface may begin to interfere with smooth joint movement. People may experience a knee "getting stuck" while climbing stairs, or a grinding in the hip. Such events can be an early warning sign of osteoarthritis.

As the disease progresses, more cartilage breaks down. The joint space narrows, and eventually, instead of effortlessly gliding over one

FIGURE 3-5: *The Progressive Development of Osteoarthritis*

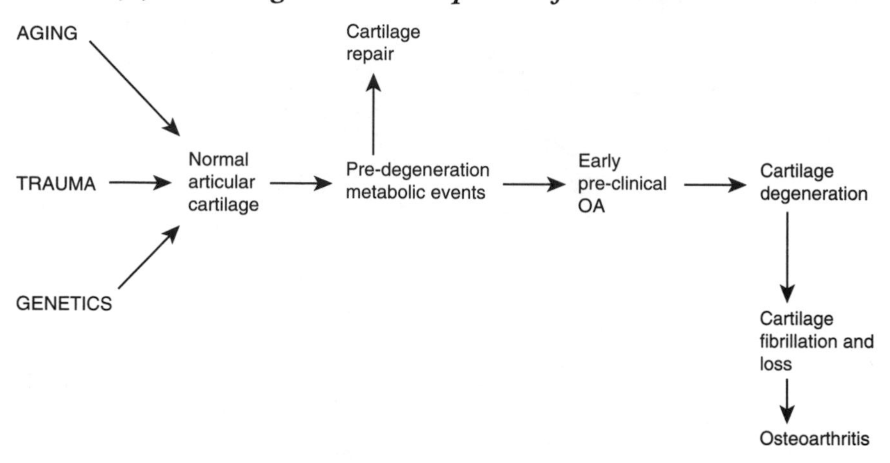

The initiating factor for osteoarthritis may be one of many things, including trauma, aging, or genetic predisposition. There is an initial breakdown of the extracellular matrix, to which the chondrocytes will respond. These cells will attempt to repair the damaged cartilage, and the repair may be successful. The attempts at repair may, however, be unsuccessful, and the incremental breakdown will become overwhelming. Ultimately the cartilage will undergo dramatic degeneration leading to osteoarthritis. These events may occur over many years.

another, bones rub on uncushioned bones, making joint motion excruciatingly painful and often totally impossible. Fortunately it usually takes many years for the process to become noticeable or to interfere with a pleasurable lifestyle.

Because osteoarthritis involves deterioration of the cartilage, the disease is often called degenerative joint disease, or DJD. Figure 3-5 schematizes the vicious cycle characteristic of osteoarthritis.

Even though osteoarthritis only involves one or a few joints—a hip, a knee, fingers, the lower back—the nonfunctioning joint often disrupts the painless movement of the entire body. Muscles distant from the affected joint may tighten in an attempt to avoid pain or spare the diseased limb. Unaffected joints may work overtime. The cartilage in an osteoarthritic knee may have worn away unevenly, thereby affecting the structure of the tibia. Eventually the entire lower leg may be deformed.

WHO SUFFERS FROM OSTEOARTHRITIS?

According to the Arthritis Foundation, 15.8 million Americans suffer from osteoarthritis, although scientists have never completely agreed on whom to include in this census. The figure should probably be higher because it does not include many who suffer some joint discomfort but do not consult a physician about these symptoms. Also, past a certain age, almost everybody's joints show some degeneration as evidenced on X rays. Persons with X-ray changes who do not have any clinical symptoms of the disease are not included in the count of osteoarthritis sufferers. Finally, many people may have early osteoarthritis, but present techniques are not sensitive enough to detect such early stages.

Even though the cause of osteoarthritis is not known, it often can and does follow overuse or injury of a particular joint. One commonly speaks of a housemaid's or a football player's knee, a bowler's thumb, a bus driver's shoulder, or a coal miner's spine. Pneumatic drill operators often develop arthritis of the wrist, and keypunch operators are prone to arthritis of the index finger. Ballerinas are at risk of developing OA of the big toe or of the hip. People who are overweight tend to have osteoarthritic knees more often than their slimmer age-mates. Right-handed people seem to have more severe OA of the right hand than those who are left-handed.

Osteoarthritis occurs in both men and women, though there are three times more women than men counted as patients. Some forms of osteoarthritis appear to be hereditary.

The prevalence of osteoarthritis is constant throughout the world indicating that neither climate nor diet play a vital role. Patients suffering from osteoarthritis, however, feel better when the weather is warm and dry rather than cold, wet, and clammy.

WHICH JOINTS ARE AFFECTED

Osteoarthritis most often affects weight-bearing joints such as the hips, knees, and spine, as shown in Figure 2-1. In the hands it attacks the joint closest to the fingertips, the middle finger joint and the joint at the base of the thumb. When OA strikes the feet, it usually affects the joint at the base of the big toe, which develops a bunion. Osteoarthritis usually spares the ankles, wrists, and elbows.

The Future

Important goals of ongoing research in osteoarthritis are slowing the disease's progress, halting it, and reversing the existing damage.

One promising approach is the recent discovery that some pharmaceutical agents can affect articular cartilage. Most agents now used for the treatment of osteoarthritis only relieve pain, decrease swelling, or provide other symptomatic relief. Newer drugs, however, might possibly influence the osteoarthritic process itself. The effectiveness of such potential drugs rests on the ability to detect osteoarthritis at a very early stage, earlier than is now routinely feasible. Diagnostic techniques such as magnetic resonance imaging (MRI) and new specific blood tests for early identification are appearing on the horizon (see Chapter 11, "The Back and Neck").

Replacement of articular cartilage destroyed by osteoarthritis is another highly attractive goal. Though cartilage can be grown in the laboratory, no tissue so far has been generated that is consistently suitable for the long-term replacement of the degenerated joint cartilage.

Other investigators study the role genetic factors play in the genesis of certain forms of osteoarthritis. While generalized osteoarthritis is extremely rare, some recent studies may shed light on the mechanisms that cause the more common forms of the disease.

◆ CHAPTER ◆

4

Pills, Pills, and More Pills

Turn on any television station and sooner or later there will be an ad for a drug that cures the "minor pains of arthritis." You sigh, because to you arthritis is no minor pain. Besides, the message is incorrect. You have tried many of the available drugs, and your arthritis is still far from cured.

As an arthritis patient you are very valuable to the drug industry. In 1993 doctors wrote millions of prescriptions for newer arthritis drugs, netting the industry approximately $2.1 billion. In 1992 over a billion more dollars were spent on nonprescription painkillers like aspirin, Tylenol, and Advil.

Since medications are an important part of arthritis treatment, you should be familiar with all aspects of your drug therapy. This chapter will teach you about the major drugs used to treat osteoarthritis, why they work, what their side effects are, and how the many available drugs differ from one another.

Medication and Osteoarthritis

Arthritis is painful, and when you consult a doctor, especially a new one, you expect to leave his or her office with a drug prescription. Chances are that you will.

As you know by now, there are as yet no medications that cure osteoarthritis. The function of the drugs prescribed for osteoarthritis is

---

WHAT TO ASK YOUR DOCTOR ABOUT THE DRUGS YOU TAKE

- *What is the name of the drug?*
- *Does the drug have a generic equivalent?*
- *How often should the medication be taken?*
- *How much should be taken?*
- *At what time of the day should the medication be taken?*
- *Should the medication be taken on an empty stomach (one hour before meals or two hours after meals), or should the medication be taken with food?*
- *How long should I take the medication?*

---

to eliminate or diminish the terrible pain characteristic of the disease. Analgesia (pain control) is, however, crucial. It is gratifying that doctors today have many options in choosing a drug that will work for you.

In deciding what drug to use first, many doctors consider not only the side effects of each drug but also the cost.

Some of the newer antiarthritis medications are very expensive; others, such as aspirin and Tylenol, cost pennies. There is also a major price difference among the newer anti-inflammatory drugs. Conscientious doctors will weigh other factors, such as the following:

- Will this patient be able to remember to take a drug several times a day, or will he or she be better off taking the drug once a day only?
- What other drugs is this patient taking?
- Has the newest drug received much publicity in the popular press? If so, would this patient be reassured if I prescribed the newest available drug?

You can help your doctor by telling him or her which prescription medication you are taking. Mention all the other drugs you take for diabetes, high blood pressure, allergy, or heart disease. Include

- ***Should the prescription be refilled if it runs out before my next appointment?***
- ***What side effects does the medication have? Does it produce stomach irritation, grogginess, sleepiness, other?***
- ***Does it interfere with driving?***
- ***What about drinking wine, beer, or liquor?***
- ***Does the medication interfere with nonprescription drugs like aspirin, acetaminophen, laxatives, etc.?***
- ***Is there anything else special about this medication?***

over-the-counter (OTC) drugs that you are taking on your own. Drugs very often interfere with one another, and the time at which you take each must be carefully adjusted. Since one often forgets drug names, many patients bring all their medications with them to the doctor's office. The box above suggests questions you should ask about each new medication.

How to Talk About Drugs

Your doctor or pharmacist may talk about generic equivalents, over-the-counter (OTC) agents, proprietary drugs, or prescription drugs. Here is what this means:

In general all drugs have

- a *chemical name,* which describes the chemical nature of the drug (the chemical name for aspirin is acetylsalicylic acid)
- a *generic* (common) name (ibuprofen and indomethacin are generic names)
- a *trade or brand name,* which is the name given by the pharmaceutical company that developed and/or manufactures the

drug (Motrin is Upjohn's trade name for ibuprofen; Indocin is Merck's trade name for indomethacin; aspirin, now a household word, is the original trade name for acetylsalicylic acid manufactured by Bayer)

At first all newly developed drugs are *proprietary* and *patented,* and are sold by the drug company that developed them. These drugs are usually expensive because there is no competition.

After a number of years, the patent protecting the drug expires, and other drug companies can manufacture it. Some companies create their own trade name for their generic equivalents; many simply use the generic name of the drug. Thus, instead of buying Indocin from Merck, you can buy indomethacin capsules from Lederle or Novopharm. These generic equivalents are usually cheaper.

Drugs are either *prescription* drugs or *nonprescription* (*over-the-counter, OTC*) drugs. OTC drugs can be bought without a doctor's prescription. For a variety of historical reasons, aspirin, an excellent drug for the treatment of the common symptoms of arthritis, is an OTC medication. Acetaminophen (Tylenol) is another. Two of the newer NSAIDs (ibuprofen and naproxen) are now OTC drugs.

Drugs Used for the Treatment of Osteoarthritis

Three types of drugs are commonly used for the treatment of osteoarthritis:

aspirin and its close relatives

acetaminophen (Tylenol, others)

newer, aspirinlike nonsteroidal anti-inflammatory drugs (NSAIDs)

Very rarely the doctor may prescribe phenylbutazone or a mild narcotic like Darvon or codeine. These drugs are excellent at relieving pain. Doctors are reluctant to prescribe them because patients who use them regularly may become addicted.

Occasionally, an individual joint may be treated with a long-acting injection of corticosteroids.

Your choice of drug should be governed by the advice of your physician, the cost of the drug, your other health problems, and most of all your individual reaction to the drug. Even though all NSAIDs are close relatives, you may tolerate some better than others.

Aspirin, the First Miracle Drug

Good drugs that alleviate the pain and stiffness of arthritis have been around for a long time. The story of aspirin begins in eighteenth-century England, where arthritis was as common as it is today. At that time people believed in the Doctrine of Signatures, which held that nature provides a cure near where a malady commonly occurs. Since arthritis has always been associated with dampness, pharmacists looked at plants that grew in swamps. The willow tree was a good candidate. In 1758 the Reverend Edward Stone prepared an extract from its bark. He prescribed the extract for fifty patients, and it indeed reduced their pain and fever. Five years later, in 1763, Stone wrote a letter about this early "drug trial" to the Royal Society in London, then the world's foremost scientific society. Soon thereafter an Italian chemist discovered that the painkilling effect of the willow bark extract was due to salicylic acid, a chemical occurring naturally in the bark.

Salicylic acid, however, irritates the stomach, and this limited its usefulness. More than a hundred years passed before Felix Hofman, a chemist employed by Bayer, specifically searched the scientific literature for a gentler pain-relieving drug. Eventually Hofman read about acetylsalicylic acid, a close chemical relative of salicylic acid, discovered in 1853 by Charles Fredrick von Gerhardt, an Alsatian chemist. Hofman called the new drug Aspirin and was gratified when this drug eased the pain of his arthritic father. Aspirin soon became the most widely used drug in the entire world.

Aspirin is a true miracle drug. For more than a century, it has stilled fever, alleviated pain, and suppressed the inflammation characteristic of many forms of arthritis. Aspirin also slows blood coagulation and today is used to reduce the risk of heart attacks.

What Are Nonsteroidal Anti-Inflammatory Drugs (NSAIDs)?

Aspirin and its many younger relatives are called nonsteroidal anti-inflammatory drugs, or NSAIDs, for short. This mouthful of a name means that these drugs decrease inflammation without being steroids like cortisone or prednisone. The latter are powerful anti-inflammatories but have many potentially dangerous side effects. Because it is chemically related to salicylic acid, aspirin is a salicylate.

For a very long time aspirin was the only drug of its kind. Its only competitor was acetaminophen (brand name Tylenol), whose benefits and pitfalls are also reviewed here. Tylenol is not an NSAID. Then, in 1961, Merck & Company discovered indomethacin (Indocin), a NSAID-like aspirin. Since that time, many new NSAIDs have been developed. By the end of 1994, the FDA had approved about twenty drugs.

How NSAIDs Relieve Pain and Inflammation

The discovery of how aspirin and its relatives suppress pain, inflammation, and fever earned John Vane, Sune Bergstroem, and Bengt I. Samuelson the 1982 Nobel Prize for medicine—the greatest honor that can be bestowed upon an investigator.

Inflammation, fever, and even pain are the body's healthy responses to injury. All three are caused by a group of substances called prostaglandins. The hormonelike prostaglandins participate in the control of blood pressure, blood coagulation, and blood flow. Prostaglandins are also active in labor, the secretion of gastric acid by the mucosa of the stomach, and the regulation of kidney function.

Prostaglandins play a role in both inflammation and pain. By interfering with the formation of many prostaglandins, the NSAIDs are effective anti-inflammatories and painkillers. Unfortunately, by curtailing the production of prostaglandins by cells, the NSAIDs also interfere with other housekeeping functions of the body and thus have many undesirable side effects.

More About Aspirin

Because it is so ancient, aspirin is available without a prescription and is inexpensive compared to the newer NSAIDs.

Aspirin is a very potent painkiller and anti-inflammatory agent. It is still the "gold standard" against which all other arthritis drugs are measured.

Unless there are clear indications to the contrary, such as a history of ulcer disease or an allergy to aspirin, some doctors start their patients on aspirin. Other physicians prefer starting with one of the newer NSAIDs that may have fewer side effects. For patients suffering from osteoarthritis, a disease in which inflammation often plays no role, some doctors prefer starting drug therapy with a pure analgesic like acetaminophen (Tylenol), which has fewer side effects. Tylenol, which is not a gastric irritant like aspirin and the other NSAIDs, works very well for many patients.

Aspirin must be used with caution at the recommended dosage. Excessive amounts can irritate the stomach, cause ringing in the ear (tinnitus), and even cause nausea, vomiting, or diarrhea. Many different pharmaceutical companies market acetylsalicylic acid preparations. Regardless of the brand name, all these pills contain the same drug. The usual dosage of aspirin for osteoarthritis is two ordinary tablets (325 mg each), four times a day. Today many drug manufacturers make somewhat bigger "aspirins," containing 500 mg of acetylsalicylic acid. These pills are often called Arthritis-Strength Aspirin.

Like most drugs the NSAIDs are absorbed into the blood from the small intestine. In order to reduce stomach irritation, some aspirin preparations are mixed with an antacid. Such preparations are called buffered aspirin. Some aspirin preparations contain caffeine to enhance their effectiveness. Others bypass the stomach with an enteric coating; some are flavored so that the tablet or syrup tastes good (St. Joseph). Still others are engineered as slow-release preparations so that the effect of the drug lasts longer.

Acetaminophen

Before reviewing the newer NSAIDs, let us look at the second old friend of the arthritis patient: acetaminophen, a drug almost as old as aspirin and one that also is available without a prescription.

Tylenol, the best known trade name of acetaminophen, is as familiar as aspirin and as widely used for the treatment of osteoarthritis. Acetaminophen accounts for 42 percent of the money spent on OTC painkillers. Like aspirin, acetaminophen decreases pain and lowers fever. The drug, however, is not an anti-inflammatory drug and so does not suppress the inflammation characteristic of many types of arthritis.

Acetaminophen acts primarily via the central nervous system and does not interfere with the production of prostaglandins that play such an important role in arthritic inflammation. The main and most important advantage of acetaminophen is that it does not irritate the stomach. Serious side effects can, however, develop after prolonged (months or years) usage.

EXAMPLE OF AN OVER-THE-COUNTER ASPIRIN PREPARATION

(See page 50 for an explanation of how to read a drug label.)

SPECIAL MESSAGE	Arthritis-Strength Aspirin
ACTIVE INGREDIENTS	Acetylsalicylic acid, 500 mg
INACTIVE INGREDIENTS	Povidone, starch, and stearic acid
INDICATIONS	For the temporary relief of simple headaches, minor pain of arthritis, muscles aches, colds, menstrual pain, toothache, or to reduce fever.
DOSAGE	2 tablets every 4 hours as needed. Do not exceed 12 tablets in 24 hours, unless directed by physician.

Look for the words acetylsalicylic acid, salicylate, salsalate, or salsamide—all of them close relatives of aspirin. A standard dose of aspirin is 325 mg or 5 grains (Gr). Do not exceed your prescribed dose of aspirin.

Like aspirin, acetaminophen is part of many medications. Always carefully read the labels of the drugs you buy. See the chart on page 50.

Newer Nonsteroidal Anti-Inflammatory Drugs

Since 1950 the Food and Drug Administration has approved about twenty new NSAIDs that, like aspirin, suppress pain, inflammation, and fever. Like aspirin, all interfere with the body's production of prostaglandins. Though they can affect the gastrointestinal tract, they are generally easier on the stomach than aspirin. They also can be taken less often—twice a day instead of four to six times a day. These NSAIDs are also distinct enough from one another that individual patients may respond better to one than another. There is no way of predicting which one of these drugs is best for you. You, with the help of your doctor, may have to try several before finding the one that works best. Two of these newer NSAIDs, ibuprofen and naproxen, are now available as OTC preparations. The appendix provides names and additional information about the currently available NSAIDs.

Reading Drug Labels

Most of us are familiar with reading food labels and can evaluate the nutritional content of the food. Nonprescription drugs have labels that are very much like the familiar food labels. It is important to read the label to determine the drug content of the preparation you buy.

The box below explains the way to read such a label. The exact wording or order of the information presented may change from one preparation to another.

Drug Side Effects

It would be nice if drugs would simply do their job and not interfere with any other physiological processes. This is rarely the case. Aspirin and most of the other NSAIDs have side effects, some more serious than others. Remember, not every patient experiences these side effects, and even when they occur they can usually be managed successfully. The following side effects require some consideration:

Irritation of the Gastrointestinal System

Irritation of the gastrointestinal tract (heartburn, dyspepsia, nausea, vomiting, ulcers) is the major side effect of the NSAIDs. The extent of the discomfort varies from patient to patient. Some patients tolerate the drugs well; others do not. The longer you take an NSAID, the more likely you are to suffer from irritation of the gastrointestinal tract. A quarter of patients taking NSAIDs develop gastric or peptic ulcers.

This stomach irritation is attributed to the fact that the NSAIDs curtail prostaglandin production. Prostaglandins normally stimulate the production of a stomach-coating mucus.

How to Read the Label of an OTC Painkiller

SPECIAL MESSAGE	May indicate some advantage of the product such as "Arthritis Strength," "Extra Strength," "Sustained Release," or "Enteric Coated."
ACTIVE INGREDIENTS	The ingredients portion of the label includes the chemical name of active drug(s) in the preparation such as acetylsalicylic acid, acetaminophen, caffeine*, antacids, and so on. For preparations containing more than one active ingredient the agents are listed in descending order, by weight. The amount in milligrams (mg) of these agents found in each tablet is usually given here or as a separate entry.
INACTIVE INGREDIENTS**	Cellulose, starch, stearic acid, silicone, or other inert substances used to make the tablet.
INDICATIONS	The purpose for which the medication is taken: temporary relief of minor aches and pains, headaches, and fever.
WARNINGS	Explains what to watch out for: keep out of reach of children, do not use without doctor's orders, do not use during pregnancy, and so on.
DOSAGE DIRECTIONS	Suggestions about amount of drug to be taken.

* Caffeine is believed to enhance the effectiveness of some drugs.

** Substances needed to manufacture a tablet.

Renal (Kidney) Toxicity

The NSAIDs can affect the kidneys, sometimes causing reversible renal insufficiency manifesting as edema (fluid retention), electrolyte imbalance (high levels of potassium), and acute renal failure. These side effects are seen most often in older patients.

Prostaglandins are once more the cause of these side effects. The kidneys, like other organs, manufacture prostaglandins, which self-regulate their function. Curtailing prostaglandin production with NSAIDs affects kidney function. If you have kidney problems, avoid using NSAIDs.

Allergy to Drugs

Fortunately, allergy to aspirin occurs rarely. Patients suffering from asthma, hay fever, or nasal polyps are at higher risk than others. Patients intolerant of aspirin often are allergic to other NSAIDs. Allergy symptoms may include fever, rashes, hives, itching, difficulties in breathing, nausea, vomiting, swelling, and so on. Contact your doctor promptly if any of these appear.

Blood Coagulation, Anemia

The NSAIDs reduce the speed at which blood coagulates. All NSAIDs, especially aspirin, must be discontinued three weeks prior to elective surgery.

Overcoming Stomach Irritation Caused by NSAIDs

Since you may feel very much better when you take NSAIDs, it may be important to take these drugs, even when they irritate your stomach. Here are strategies that may help:

- *Taking NSAIDs with food:* In order to reduce stomach irritation, take the medication with food or soon after a meal.
- *Avoiding other stomach irritants:* Avoid or cut down on the use of alcohol, tobacco, and caffeine (coffee, tea, cola, chocolate) since these also irritate the stomach.
- *Carefully selecting your NSAID:* Aspirin is particularly hard on the stomach. Some of the newer NSAIDs are gentler. It usually takes some trial and error to find the NSAID that is best for you.
- *Use the enteric-coated medication:* These preparations are designed to release the medication in the small intestine after the tablet or capsule passes through the stomach.

- *Protecting the stomach with another drug:* Four types of medication reduce the gastrointestinal side effects of NSAIDs:
    - man-made prostaglandins
    - H-2 blockers
    - coating agents
    - antacids

Man-Made Prostaglandins: During the 1970s, when it became apparent that prostaglandins played such an important role in regulating the biological processes of the body, pharmacologists tried to synthesize man-made equivalents. Misoprostol (brand name Cytotec) is one result of their ingenuity. Like its natural counterpart, misoprostol curtails gastric acid formation and stimulates the stomach to produce gastric mucus. This dual action of misoprostol reduces the incidence of ulcers in patients taking NSAIDs.

H-2 Blockers: Cimetidine (Tagamet), ranitidine (Zantac), and other drugs that inhibit the release of stomach acid revolutionized the treatment of gastric ulcers. The drugs also enable many patients to take such stomach-irritating drugs as aspirin and other NSAIDs.

Coating Agents: Sucralfate (Carafate) physically coats existing ulcer sites, thereby protecting them from contact with acid, promoting healing, and enabling patients to take stomach-irritating medication.

Antacids: Antacids like Rolaids, Milk of Magnesia, Tums, Alka-Seltzer, Mylanta, and countless other nonprescription drugs have been used for centuries to reduce excess acid in the stomach.

How the Body Utilizes Drugs

Many of the excellent drugs available today are responsible for our good health and longevity. In order to take these drugs safely and accurately, you should understand how the body utilizes them.

Most drugs used for the treatment of osteoarthritis are taken by mouth and are absorbed into the blood from the small intestine. If they are to do their job and suppress pain and inflammation, the concentration of the drug in the blood must be above a certain level. The time it takes for these drugs to reach this concentration varies. The NSAIDs are absorbed rapidly. Most reach their peak level within the hour.

Since the body considers all medications "toxic," it also tries to get rid of them as quickly as possible. Drugs are dismantled in the liver, the body's detoxification plant, and excreted by the kidneys in the urine. The speed at which the body degrades drugs varies. Some drugs are degraded within minutes; others take hours, or even days.

Maintaining the drug at or above a necessary concentration requires balancing *the amount taken* with *its rate of elimination.* For each drug the dosage and the number of times the drug has to be taken during the day is carefully determined by the drug manufacturer.

New manufacturing methods can make short-lived drugs last longer. A few decades ago chemists found a way to engineer pills so they do not deliver their drug cargo all at once. The time-release medications were born. For instance, a medication that is quickly eliminated from the body is milled into small sprinkle-like granules. These are coated with chemicals that dissolve in body fluids at different rates. Careful measurements and decade-long experience have shown that two aspirins, taken every four hours, alleviate pain. Now there are sustained-release formulations that make an aspirin capsule last eight hours.

It is easy to understand why it is important to take all medications as prescribed. Yet detailed studies have shown that only 60 percent of all older persons take their medication as directed by their doctors. Physicians also make mistakes, prescribing too much, too little, or the wrong combination of drugs. Accurate figures are very hard to come by, but all in all, and for a variety of reasons, drug misadventures (which include adverse drug reaction, dosing errors, drug interactions, and misunderstanding of physician instructions) are responsible for approximately 10 percent of all hospital admissions!

It is very easy to forget to take your medicine or not to remember whether you have taken it. Several good pill-minders are available.

Another method is to keep a record of the pills you take. A simple calendar will do. Paste it on the wall near your bathroom mirror and make a check each time you take your medication.

Some of the information presented in this chapter may seem cumbersome. Don't be discouraged. Among the many available drugs, it is likely that several will be just right for you. They will help you to live a full life in spite of osteoarthritis.

◆ CHAPTER ◆

5

Exercise, Physical Therapy, and Osteoarthritis

The Physical Therapist

Fifty years ago doctors cautioned all patients with arthritis to take it easy and lead a sedentary life. Then it became apparent that excessive physical inactivity engenders bone and muscle loss—and today patients leave the doctor's office with an exercise prescription. Exercise is an essential part of your treatment.

There are two kinds of exercises for arthritis patients:

- therapeutic exercises to keep joints affected by osteoarthritis in as good working order as possible
- conditioning exercises to promote fitness, strengthen your muscles, and maintain body weight

You must be taught how to do the therapeutic exercises correctly. Since your body is impaired by osteoarthritis, which limits painfree movement, you may also need some help with the fitness portion of your exercise program.

The health professional in charge of all your exercises is the physical therapist. He or she may remind you of the phys-ed teacher or sports coach you had when you were a kid. He or she will teach you how to exercise and will get upset when you don't do the prescribed "homework."

In addition to a healthy respect for physical performance, physical therapists have an in-depth understanding of body mechanics. They are also aware of the limitations imposed by a degenerative disease like arthritis. Good physical therapists will never promise you more than your body can deliver. One of their tasks is to teach patients to have realistic expectations. No amount of exercise will regenerate the knee cartilage destroyed by arthritis. Strengthening the muscles that surround the knee will, however, enable many patients to have a knee functional enough for everyday use.

A patient's response to a prescribed program of therapy may help the physician decide if and when surgery is indicated. Patients whose muscle tissue is in good shape often recover more fully and more quickly than patients with long-term disuse. It is not always wise to postpone surgery as long as possible.

Often physical therapists are able to teach their patients to overcome the disabling pain of arthritis with simple exercises. Many patients are extremely grateful to their physical therapist. If you are lucky, your physical therapist may become your best friend.

TAKING RESPONSIBILITY

Terry O'Halloran, a physical therapist at Columbia Presbyterian, teaches his patients that they are responsible for their own physical well-being. Often this means lowering the patient's expectations and working slowly to improve function.

Terry specializes in rehabilitating patients after joint replacement surgery. He is equally skilled in providing exercises for patients with freshly operated hips, knees, or shoulders.

Though osteoarthritis has been around for a very long time (fossil records show dinosaurs suffered from the disease) the use of exercise to treat it is rather new. Patients used to be instructed to rest the affected joint. Today, one of the first directives given to every arthritis patient is the seemingly contradictory instruction to "rest and exercise."

Rest, which we'll talk about later, is extremely important for any patient with arthritis. Adequate sleep—including naps—restores the body and rests painful joints. Short rests between exercises allow the muscles to recover.

The Role of Exercise

Every joint depends on motion for its health and nourishment. To put it more bluntly, "Use it or lose it."

Muscles, which enable the joints to move, must be exercised regularly to stay functional. All living creatures thrive on movement, and a relatively active, normal lifestyle keeps the muscles in reasonable shape. Conversely, anyone who has ever had a limb enclosed in a cast knows how quickly inactive muscles deteriorate. Formal exercises usually play an important role in the treatment of persons suffering from musculoskeletal disorders. Arthritis and chronic back pain, for example, are aggravated by a tendency to avoid using certain muscles—often the very muscles most needed to retard joint deterioration.

It will not do, however, to force a painful arthritic joint to work hard and indiscriminately. Motion of any joint, even a healthy one, should never be abusive. People suffering from arthritis must select the exercises they do very carefully. Exercises that are extremely beneficial for one person may be harmful for another. Exercises must be treated like medication; physical therapists and other exercise experts teach patients how to do them properly.

The Pain Cycle

It is easy to see how movement eliminates pain. We are all familiar with the discomfort of an arm or a foot that "goes to sleep." Gentle motion restores blood flow and abolishes pain. Something similar happens with arthritis. Almost every arthritis patient is stiff in the morning or after prolonged immobility. Standing, stretching, or taking a hot bath remedies that condition.

The natural reaction to pain is avoidance of pain. In the case of joints this means avoiding using the particular joint (disuse). When prolonged, this results in muscle tightness and loss of motion. Progressive joint contracture and stiffness continue to perpetuate this cycle. Figure 5-1 (page 58) illustrates the circle of pain and loss of mobility.

FIGURE 5-1: *The Vicious Circle: Pain and Loss of Mobility*

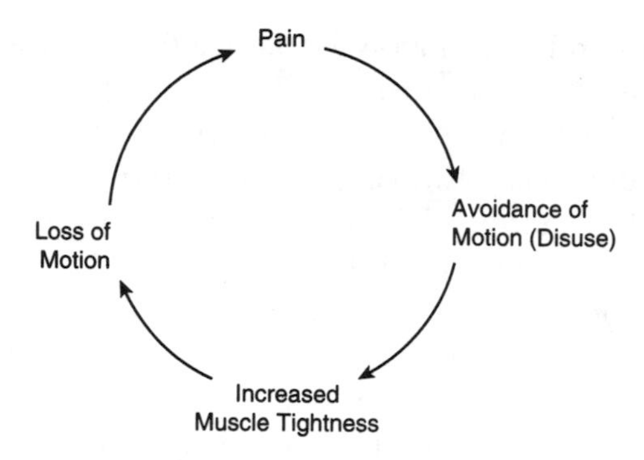

ASSESSMENT

No physical therapist will start you on an exercise program without

- carefully reviewing your medical history
- checking with your physician
- personally evaluating you

During the assessment physical therapists will evaluate the flexibility and length of your muscles. To evaluate your hamstrings they have you bend over. Can you touch your toes? For other muscles they have you reach behind your back with your arms, or try to touch your buttocks with your heel. Directing you to walk, stand, and walk again, they study your posture and gait. Recently physical therapists have started videotaping their patients as they walk or run. When these films are played back slowly and analyzed, the therapist can often pinpoint particular problems.

TYPES OF EXERCISES

The goal of exercise is to

- Improve joint function by
    - maintaining the mobility of a joint
    - maintaining the correct alignment of a joint
    - strengthening the muscles surrounding the joint

- maintain or improve cardiovascular function
- maintain or decrease body weight
- improve overall muscle tone
- prevent osteoporosis

Three types of exercises are prescribed to achieve these goals:

- range of motion exercises
- strengthening exercises
- aerobic (conditioning) exercises

The name of each type of exercise is self-explanatory. The goal of the range of motion or stretching exercises is to maintain the natural movement of a joint. Joint mobility naturally decreases with age, and it is important for everyone to take each joint through its full range of motion daily.

Range of motion exercises are further subdivided into *active* and *passive*. Active movements are those you can do on your own—for instance, turning your hip outward when you lie on your back or curling up your index finger. Passive movements need the addition of assistance from another person or another part of your body. Pushing down your index finger with the other hand is an example of a passive exercise; someone bending your knee is another.

Your Exercise Program

Your doctor or physical therapist will provide you with a written list of exercises that focus on your particular needs. The physical therapist will watch you do these exercises to make sure you are doing them correctly. Then you will do them alone, at home.

You may see the physical therapist for several sessions in a row. Some patients return to their physical therapist after a couple of months to make sure that the exercises are still being done properly. Improperly done exercises can actually be counterproductive. Such follow-up sessions, however, are not always paid for by health insurance.

Preparation for Exercise

Schedule your exercises as faithfully as you plan your meals. Have a specific place where you do them. You may wish to do your exercises in front of a full-length mirror, play music, or turn on a favorite television program. If necessary, take your analgesic (Tylenol, aspirin, NSAIDs) so that its effect is maximum before you work out. Always warm up before you exercise.

Warming Up

"Cold" muscles, like cold taffy, won't stretch. You may increase blood flow to the tissues by taking a hot shower or bath, or by applying a warm, moist Turkish towel.

Always start your exercises by stretching every part of your body. You can do some of that lying in bed or sitting.

Visualize your entire body and limber it up from top to bottom.

How to Exercise

- Have an exercise specialist show you how to do an exercise. Then do the exercise while the expert is watching.
- Start exercising slowly, at low intensity. Ask your therapist what discomfort to expect and when to stop exercising.
- Do your exercises regularly. Twenty minutes a day is fine; thirty is even better.
- Exercise whenever you hurt least.

Range-of-Motion Exercises

Figure 5-2 shows some range-of-motion exercises or stretching exercises (see warning on page 62). The Arthritis Foundation recommends these steps:

1. Do these exercises once or twice daily to maintain joint mobility. Repeat each exercise five to ten times.
2. Move in a slow, steady manner. Do not bounce.
3. Stretch gently at the end of each motion, but not so far that you are in pain.
4. Breathe regularly as you exercise. DO NOT HOLD YOUR BREATH. You may want to count out loud.

FIGURE 5-2: *Sample Range-of-Motion Exercises*

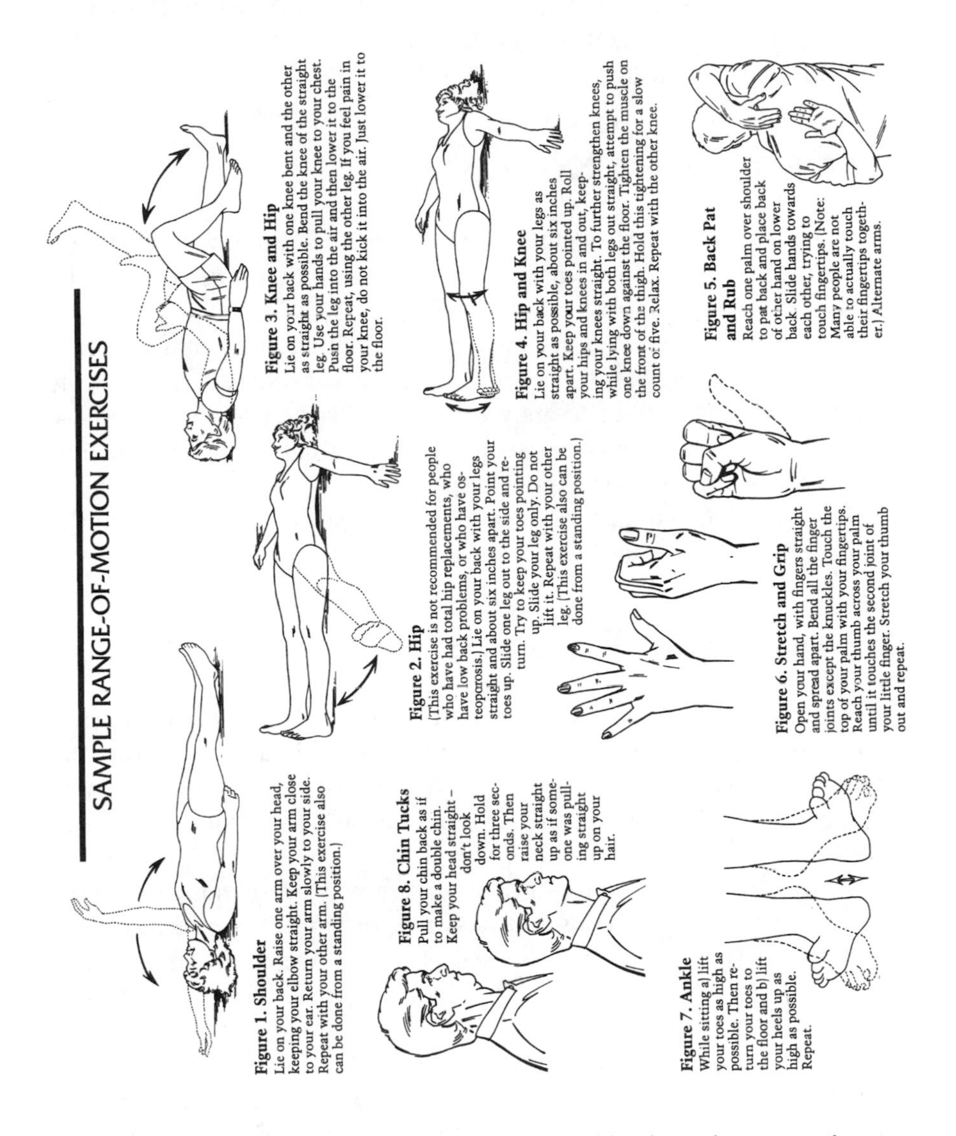

These basic range-of-motion exercises are suggested by the Arthritis Foundation. *Reprinted with permission from the Arthritis Foundation.*

DO THE EXERCISES DESCRIBED ON PAGE 60 ONLY IF YOU HAVE NO ACTIVE MUSCULOSKELETAL PROBLEM. IF YOU ARE UNDER MEDICAL CARE, ASK YOUR PHYSICIAN ABOUT THE APPROPRIATENESS OF THE EXERCISES.

Strengthening Exercises

These are designed to strengthen the muscles surrounding joints, thereby permitting better joint movement. Strengthening exercise can be either isometric or isotonic.

During isometric exercise, muscles are tightened (contracted) and released without moving the joint. This kind of exercise is particularly useful when it is painful to move the joint. During isotonic exercise muscles are moved against resistance such as a light weight or against the resistance of your own body weight.

Strengthening exercise must be done, at least to begin with, under the supervision of a therapist.

Conditioning Exercises

Conditioning or aerobic exercises improve overall physical health, especially heart and lung function, and help you maintain an appropriate body weight. To be effective they have to be done for at least twenty minutes three times a week. This is why they are also called endurance exercises.

Thirty years ago, when John F. Kennedy was president, it suddenly dawned on the nation's consciousness that urbanization and motorization left Americans in poor physical shape. Since then America has been on an exercise kick. Parks are full of joggers and bikers, and exercise gyms are a growth industry.

People with arthritis may not be able to jog, play tennis, or score in touch football, but most can find an enjoyable physical activity they can do alone or with others. With careful study and prudent experimentation, you can judge what kind of activity is good for you. As a rule, choose an exercise that spares your arthritic joints, and one in which impact is minimal. Do not persist with a sport that you dislike or one that causes pain either during its performance or after you are finished. Table 5-1 gives an overview of suitable exercises. Remember

TABLE 5-1: ***Sports Activities Suitable for Patients with Osteoarthritis***

If the Arthritis Affects	You Can Do
upper extremities (shoulders, elbows)	swimming, running, cross-country skiing, hiking, walking, bicycling, aquatic exercises
back, cervical spine	swimming, aquatic exercises
lower extremities (hips, knees, ankles)	swimming, aquatic exercises, rowing, golfing, stationary bicycling, canoeing, water running

that everyone is unique. Check with your physician before actually beginning or continuing an exercise program or investing in an exercise machine.

Sports for People with Arthritis

Having to abandon a special sport because of joint impairment is emotionally disturbing and deprives your body of the essential benefits of that exercise. Here is a look at some common sports, with suggestions on how to adapt them to your needs. For every sport, you are the best judge of whether the activity is pleasurable or not.

Walking and hiking are among the best all-around conditioning exercises. Both can, however, be a problem if arthritis affects your the weight-bearing joints. Interrupting the activity with frequent rest periods may be helpful.

Swimming avoids stressing weight-bearing joints. It also relaxes the muscles, decreases pain, and permits moving joints without impact. Those who can't swim can still paddle around in the water with water wings, in a tube, or by hanging on to a kickboard. Cold water may be a problem for patients suffering from arthritis, but many YMCAs, YWCAs, and private health clubs maintain water temperatures appropriate for therapeutic swimming. Persons suffering from degeneration of the cervical spine should check with their physician about swimming.

Many joggers derive a special high from running. When arthritis interferes with running, you may be able to "jog" in a pool. An Aquajogger buoyancy belt enables swimmers, and even nonswimmers, to run in the water and reap the pleasures and benefits of jogging without stressing the weight-bearing joints. Aquajoggers are available from sports equipment stores and catalogues. (For example: Self-Care, 5850 Shellmound Street, Emeryville, CA 94662-0813. Tel: 800-345-3371.)

Water aerobics, which are discussed later in this chapter, are an ideal substitute for the more traditional variety of these exercises.

If you were a downhill skier who mourns the exhilaration of winter, snow, and cold weather, you may be able to settle for gentler cross-country skiing. Skiing, always associated with a certain amount of falling and an increased risk of broken bones, is not recommended for those who have undergone total hip or knee-joint replacement surgery.

Golf is good exercise for the arm and shoulder joints and offers natural rest periods. The sport can, however, be tough for those suffering from an arthritic lower back. Golfers should not caddy their own clubs, however.

Bicycling is good exercise. It may be enjoyable for some and painful for others. Biking on flat ground without resistance is fine. Strenuous, uphill biking is not indicated for those with osteoarthritis of the hips or knees.

Actual rowing and canoeing are excellent exercises for those who suffer from arthritis of the hips and knees. A rowing machine, however, usually puts too much stress on these joints.

Depending on how you play tennis, it can be a good form of exercise. If you run and jump a lot, it is not for you. Pain is a good indicator of what you can and cannot do.

Exercise Machines for People with Arthritis

The new and widely available exercise machines exercise most joints. The most useful of these are stationary bicycles, rowing machines, skiing machines, and treadmills. These machines can be used at gyms or bought for home use.

The *stationary bicycle* is the most widely used home exercise machine. It mostly exercises the leg muscles, but provides adequate cardiovascular fitness conditioning. Care must be taken to select a model in which the resistance can be easily adjusted. This is especially important for those suffering from OA of the knees. More expensive stationary bicycles provide all kinds of refinements such as automatic tension adjustment to simulate uphill and downhill biking, heart rate monitoring, and calories used per unit of time.

Rowing machines provide excellent overall conditioning of the skeletal and abdominal muscles. Like bicycling, rowing is non-weight-bearing. However, it entails a lot of hip and knee bending and may not be suitable for people suffering from osteoarthritis of the hips and knees.

Skiing machines improve skeletal muscle tone of the legs, arms, and back, and provide aerobic conditioning. Two types of ski machines are currently available, the classic "Nordic" machine and an easier-to-use "cross-country" model equipped with ski poles.

Treadmills, especially the mechanical ones with rolling surfaces and elevation control, can be expensive, but even less expensive models provide a good workout for people who have no trouble walking.

The effects of *weight lifting* can be simulated by a variety of machines that strengthen individual muscle groups. These machines, available in many gyms, are extremely popular.

Videotapes

One of the best ways to do both range-of-motion and strengthening exercises is to work out with videotapes. The Arthritis Foundation, through its PACE (People with Arthritis Can Exercise) programs, offers tapes for people with both moderate and severe arthritis. Tapes can be ordered from your local chapter or by calling 1-800-933-0032.

How to Select an Exercise Program

The key to a successful exercise program is to choose an activity that does not aggravate your arthritis, is enjoyable, is affordable, and fits your time schedule and your athletic skill. Before selecting an activity, check with your physician and consider the following:

What Kind of Osteoarthritis Do You Have? To a large extent, your disease dictates what type of sport or exercise you can participate in. Many people manage to carry on with their favorite sport in spite of their arthritis. Downhill skiers may switch to cross-country. Tennis players may play doubles instead of singles, joggers may race-walk or take long rambles.

How Physically Fit Are You? If you've been physically inactive for a while, you may want to start slowly with brisk walking or swimming rather than jogging or jumping rope.

How Old Are You? Remember, nobody is ever too old to exercise. Provided the exercise program is tailored to the appropriate fitness level, middle-aged and older people benefit from regular physical activity just as much as young people do.

People who have not exercised for a while, however, should start with mild exercise. During the initial few months gradually build the length and intensity of the exercise session. If you are over sixty, walking and swimming are especially suitable.

Do You Like to Exercise Alone or with Others? Select your exercise program accordingly. Pick a team sport, a two-person activity, or something you can do alone like swimming. Companionship may help you get started and keep you going. Today many communities have walking clubs.

Where Do You Prefer to Exercise? Outdoor activities offer a variety of scenery. Indoor activities offer protection from the weater. It is often advantageous to have one outdoor and one indoor activity.

How Much Money Can You Spend? Some exercises and sports require expensive equipment or membership fees. Others, such as walking or bicycling, are inexpensive.

How Much Time Do You Have? Some exercises, especially those which require partners or a trip to the gym, are rather time-consuming. Others, like switching on an exercise tape or cycling on a stationary bike, only take twenty to thirty minutes a day. Regardless of the time you plan to spend, make exercise a regular part your day.

How Athletic Are You? Select an activity that you can master. You will not want to continue with a sport when the activity is frustrating.

How to Maintain an Exercise Program

It is easier to start an exercise program than to maintain it week after week and month after month. Yet all the benefits of exercise—

cardiovascular fitness, weight loss, strengthening of muscle tone—are predicated on *doing exercise regularly.*

TIPS ON HOW TO MAINTAIN AN EXERCISE PROGRAM*

Avoiding Boredom: Doing anything three or four times a week becomes tedious. It may be helpful to exercise with a partner or join a club. During solitary, stationary exercise (cycling, rowing, skiing) you can read a book or watch television.

Exercise tapes, many of them designed to be used with a specific exercise machine, are most helpful. Two sources are Cyclovision Tours, which stocks eleven different tapes for stationary bicycles, six for cross-country skiing, and three for stair-stepping (800-624-4952), and Collage Video, which stocks 280 different exercise videos, including some designed especially for arthritis patients (800-433-6769).

Lack of Time: Finding time for exercise is difficult, especially if you go to work or run a busy household. Sometimes you can integrate exercise with your regular activities—exercising while listening to the news, walking instead of driving, or taking the stairs instead of the elevator. Sometimes you just have to take the time.

Avoiding Discomfort and Injury: Arthritis hurts, and you may be reluctant to increase the discomfort by exercising. Plan your exercise sessions for when you hurt least—after a hot bath or when your pain medication is maximally effective.

Listen to your body, which may tell you that you exercise too hard. It is important to start exercising slowly to avoid fatigue and muscle pain. If you exercise outdoors, dress according to the weather. On hot days drink lots of water. On cold days wear layered clothes that can be taken off, mittens or gloves, and a hat (40 percent of the body's heat is lost through the head and neck). On rainy, icy, or snowy days be aware of reduced visibility and slippery pathways. Do not exercise for two hours after a heavy meal, and rest your arthritic joints after exercising vigorously. Wear comfortable shoes with good soles and adequate cushioning.

*Some of the information is adapted from *Exercise and Your Heart:* NIH Publication # 81-1677.

Aquatics Programs

Warm water does wonders for people suffering from arthritis. Many patients do extremely well performing exercises in a warm, shallow swimming pool. Water endows the body with buoyancy and reduces stress on the joints, making all exercises, including the all-important range-of-motion exercises, much easier. The water feels good, and simply being in a warm swimming pool provides relaxation, improves mobility, and decreases pain. The aqua exercises should, however, be as carefully prescribed as those performed on dry land to ensure that performing them will keep the joints as mobile as possible.

The Arthritis Foundation runs aquatic exercise programs at YMCAs and YWCAs throughout the United States.

A typical class takes place in a warm pool around 83° F with soft music in the background. Exercise instructions are simple and easy to follow: "Stand on one leg, point the toes . . . use your foot as if you were cleaning off your shoes . . . shuffle in the sand . . . hold on to the wall, open and close your legs thirty times as if they were pulled by a rubber band. Inhale, get tall—exhale—shrink . . . take the water wings and pump them in the water up and down, use your arms as if you were to pick up the water. . . . "

Because most participants suffer from longstanding arthritis and have attended classes for a long time, they often need little instruction. The aquatics programs cater to a loyal clientele.

The Arthritis Foundation/YMCA Aquatics Program (AFYAP) is open to all adults suffering from arthritis. Call your local chapter of the Arthritis Foundation for details. The Arthritis Foundation also sells a videotape which demonstrates fifty different pool exercises. This tape can be ordered by calling 800-497-6137.

Reducing the Risk of Sports-Induced Injuries

Sports enthusiasts have a tendency to overdo things, including all forms of exercise. As jogging and other sports became more popular, orthopedists and physical therapists began to see more people suffering from overuse syndromes.

Most often these people needed to learn moderation, muscle stretching and strengthening, and the difference between sports and exercise. Because many sports strengthen some muscle groups but not others, the body is often not fully toned. In addition to doing their chosen sport, many active people have to learn to exercise their unused muscles. This can easily be done by varying the exercise routine—for instance, running one day and working out at the gym the next.

Posture

Much musculoskeletal grief comes from the way we do things. We slump in our chairs, shuffle and slouch when we walk, don't bend our knees when we pick up objects off the floor, sleep on a soft mattress. Here are some suggestions on how to improve posture and keep the body balanced:

Standing

- Wear comfortable shoes. Walking sneakers are ideal. Widen your base of support by keeping your feet shoulder-width apart.
- Stand as straight as you can. Tuck in your stomach and buttocks; keep your shoulders down.
- When standing for a long time, rest one foot on a chair rung, stool, or other elevated surface. Alternate feet every few minutes.
- Use a cane if so advised by your physician or physical therapist.

Sitting

- Sit on a dining-room-height chair with a straight back rather than a lounge chair.
- Rest both feet on the floor, and if they don't reach, use a footstool. Keep your knees at right angles, or better still, higher than your hips.

- When working at a desk, make sure it is high enough in relation to your chair so that you do not hunch over.
- Get up often—every twenty minutes or so—and move about.
- Make sure your spine is supported. A back rest (available in many mail order catalogs or surgical supply stores) or a rolled towel inserted at the height of the small of the back prevents backache.
- The Scandinavian chairs that make you "sit on your knees" can be extremely relaxing for the back.

Driving

- Sit far enough front to keep your knees higher than your hips.
- Use a back rest or small rolled towel to support your lower back.
- Stop at least once an hour. Walk around and stretch.

Sleeping

- Sleep on a firm mattress.
- Sleep on your side or back with knees bent and a small pillow in between your legs or under your knees.

Lifting

- Avoid lifting. If you must lift, use your legs, not your back. Kneel with one leg to pick up load.
- Keep load as close to your body as possible.

CANES

If you have arthritis of the weight-bearing joints, you'd be surprised at the pain relief provided by a simple cane or walker. If you have an arthritic hip, carry the cane in the opposite hand; otherwise use the cane in either hand.

Your physical therapist or the salesman at a good surgical supply store will adjust the height of your cane. To be the proper height, the wrist of the hand that holds the cane should be at the height of the cane's head.

You may find it useful to own a folding cane. It can travel in your pocket book and emerge, when necessary, during long shopping, museum, or sight-seeing trips.

◆ CHAPTER ◆

6

Rehabilitation and Pain Management

Martha B. looked at her doctor's latest prescription for the newest non-steroidal anti-inflammatory drug. She knew that it would not quell her pain for long. She'd give it a try, but . . .

Many patients suffering from osteoarthritis have a similar experience. Drugs alone are not the answer to coping with chronic pain. Fortunately there are other ways. Patients who cope well with their disease do so because they have learned to deal with the pain and depression associated with chronic musculoskeletal disease.

This chapter presents a grab bag of time-tested pain-relief techniques. Some of these will work for you, others not. Living well in spite of osteoarthritis, however, is a very worthwhile endeavor, and exploring ways of pain control makes sense.

The Rehabilitation Specialist

Rehabilitation specialists, also known as physiatrists, approach patients in a unique manner. Traditionally doctors look at their patients in terms of what the patient can't do. Physiatrists find out what their patients *can do,* and then maximize this potential.

Louis S. Halstead, from Baylor College of Medicine, explains that, in contrast to traditional doctors, rehabilitation specialists view themselves as teachers and facilitators and believe in active patient participation through a team approach.

Their treatment goals are to help patients heal, cope, adjust, and enhance their functional performance.

To accomplish these goals, rehabilitation specialists rely heavily on such traditional modalities as heat, cold, massage, rest, and other physical measures that relieve pain. They work closely with occupational and physical therapists, two health professionals who play a major role in the treatment of osteoarthritis. An occupational therapist teaches patients to perform specific tasks, such as tying shoes or keeping house with ease, in spite of a particular physical impairment. (Also see Chapter 13.)

Diagnosis

You have already gathered that each member of the arthritis team does his or her own diagnostic evaluation. Physiatrists spend a lot of time listening to their patients and also rely on newer techniques like CT-scans and MRIs (magnetic resonance imaging), as well as traditional X rays.

As a rule, physicians refer patients to physiatrists only if their condition has not responded to standard therapy. It is hoped that the physiatrist will be able to suggest specific treatment approaches and provide encouragement, counseling, and support. Ultimately, if this approach is successful, the patient will be his or her own therapist, performing many of the suggested therapies at home.

For patients with chronic pain, diagnosis is especially important. These patients usually have taken a whole host of medications, including NSAIDs and tranquilizers such as Valium, which at best have only been partially satisfactory. The rehabilitation specialist spends a lot of time reviewing the past medical history of the patient. Lifestyle and home and working environment are evaluated carefully.

Once identified, the solution may be simple. Perhaps the pain is the result of occupational stresses like excessive lifting, standing, stair climbing, and driving. Rearrangement of working conditions may enable this patient to return to a normal, pleasurable life.

A Commitment to Therapy

Most patients and physicians want instant results. With chronic pain therapy this is not possible. Before consulting a physiatrist, it is important for patients to realize that it is unlikely that any single treatment will control the pain. Nor will it be enough to try each treatment once.

Pain and the Chronic Pain Syndrome

Everyone is familiar with pain: its alleviation is probably medicine's oldest and most continuous quest. Our distant ancestors discovered the opiates, which are still among the most potent commonly used analgesics. Even aspirin, the wonder drug, was discovered more than one hundred years ago, although natural salicylates were used by primitive people much earlier.

To begin with, pain is a protective mechanism telling the body that something is wrong. For musculoskeletal diseases like osteoarthritis, pain urges the body to stop using the affected joint.

Most often pain is self-limited. It ceases without treatment when its cause disappears. Some arthritis patients, unfortunately, must deal with chronic pain. In such cases, while the inflammation that caused the initial pain has subsided, the disease process has damaged nerves or soft tissues, resulting in a new, chronic, or continuous pain.

The Relief of Chronic Pain

The Princess and the Pea

In one of his beloved fairy tales, Hans Christian Andersen tells of the queen who hid a pea under one hundred mattresses to make sure that the girl who wanted to marry her son was indeed a princess. The next morning, when asked how she had slept, the girl declared she was black and blue and had not slept a wink. The queen was satisfied, and let her son wed the girl, for only a princess would be sensitive enough to feel a pea through one hundred mattresses. (Today's experts would have pointed out that one hundred soft mattresses, alone, without the pea, surely will cause a severe backache!)

Like Andersen's princess, we all have different pain thresholds and respond individually to pain relief measures. Here is a series of suggestions on how to alleviate pain. You may have to try all or most of them to find what works for you. (Some of these suggestions were inspired by the Arthritis Foundation's booklet "Coping with Pain.")

Attitude

Sure, her back hurts, but Mary won't let that stop her from going to her grandchild's birthday party. She'll lie down for a rest before she goes, then she'll take a hot shower, an extra aspirin, and her cane.

Mary did have a good time, better than Anna, Joanna's other grandmother, who decided to stay home with her hurting hip and feel sorry for herself. Mary was also better off than Theresa, who insisted on going to the party early to help with preparations, though her knee was killing her. Mary, Anna, and Theresa are imaginary characters, but they are good examples of how to live with pain. Pain requires its due. Patients who acknowledge their discomfort yet deal with it sensibly are much better off than those who deny its existence or let it rule their lives.

Drug Therapy

Pain-relieving medications (analgesics) are a crucial adjunct in the treatment of osteoarthritis. Chapter 4 extensively discusses their use. For continuous pain relief, it is important to take such drugs only as directed. In fact, doctors often discourage their chronic pain patients from using narcotic and other addictive medications because patients can build up a tolerance to these drugs—leading to larger and larger doses, which provide less and less pain relief. This leaves the patient with a problem more serious than the original condition.

Heat

One of the most effective ways of relieving arthritic pain is through the simple application of either superficial or deep heat. As the names imply, each affects different layers of tissue. Both types of heat

- decrease joint stiffness
- lessen pain

- relieve muscle spasm
- increase blood flow

Superficial Heat

Every arthritis patient knows the relief provided by a hot bath, an electric blanket, or an electrically heated mattress pad. The familiar hot water bottle provides more localized heat.

Since hot water bottles cool very quickly, patients are tempted to use electric heating pads. Be careful to turn these off before falling asleep, and never put the heating pad under the treated area. Lying on the pad reduces air and local blood circulation, and even at low temperatures the accumulated heat can cause serious burns.

Nobody knows quite why, but moist heat is often more effective for treating musculoskeletal pain than dry heat. It is easy to prepare a moist heat pack at home.

One easy way of preparing a hot pack is to soak a Turkish towel in water and heat it in the microwave at medium heat for three minutes or so. Drugstores sell a variety of compresses that retain heat for twenty to thirty minutes. One such claylike preparation, called a hydrocollator, is heated in boiling water.

All compresses should be comfortably warm but not scalding hot. Nevertheless, always protect your skin with a cloth or towel before applying the heat pack. Apply the compress for about twenty minutes. Paraffin baths (see Chapter 13) provide relief for patients suffering from arthritis of the hands or feet.

Deep Heat

Heat delivered directly over the involved area often relieves the pain long enough for patients to perform range-of-motion exercises. In these techniques different forms of energy are converted to heat deep inside the body. The two most commonly used techniques for arthritis patients are diathermy and ultrasound.

Unlike superficial heat, which can be applied by the patient at home, deep heat application is an office procedure requiring a skilled therapist. A typical treatment lasts fifteen to thirty minutes.

During any of these procedures, the therapist will position you in a chair or on a table, so that he or she has easy access to the joint. Relax—none of these procedures hurt.

Diathermy transforms shortwave radiation into deep heat. Since the radiation concentrates in metal, diathermy is contraindicated for patients with metallic surgical implants, such as a total hip. Care must also be taken to remove all metallic jewelry and clothing with metal fasteners before initiating therapy.

Ultrasound equipment delivers high-energy sound waves, which also convert to heat. Metal as such does not interfere, but ultrasound may overheat and possibly weaken the methylmethacrylate glue used to cement prostheses in place. Make sure you tell your therapist if any of this applies to you.

One advantage of ultrasound therapy is that the amount of heat delivered to deeper joint areas can be controlled. In addition to improved joint function, ultrasound may have a beneficial effect on connective tissue. It often mobilizes a "frozen" joint or relieves muscle contractures.

The ultrasound treatment begins with the application of conducting gel. Then the therapist moves the ultrasound head back and forth over the joint.

Microwaves are also used for deep heat therapy. However, since microwaves accumulate in tissues with a high water content, microwave diathermy is not terribly useful for the treatment of bones and deep joint tissue, although it is effective for muscle problems.

Cold

"Try heat, and if it doesn't work, try ice," is the surprising message you may receive from many therapists. Like other methods of pain relief, the benefit one derives from either is highly individual. Cold has a numbing effect that is most helpful for acutely inflamed joints. Cold initially causes vasoconstriction (narrowing of the blood vessels), followed by vasodilation (widening of the blood vessels, which in turn increases the blood supply). Heat causes only vasodilation.

Cold can be supplied by an ice bag or by wrapping ice cubes or frozen vegetables in a towel. ElastoGel Hot/Cold wraps are a more modern method, supplying cold for twenty to forty minutes when frozen, or heat for twenty to thirty minutes when heated in the microwave. These wraps, shaped for necks, shoulders, ankles, or knees, are available in sports shops or from catalogs.

Hydrotherapy

The use of baths to relieve pain is an old remedy. A hot bath or shower is still one of the easiest ways of decreasing pain, relieving muscle spasms, improving range of motion, and providing relaxation. Very hot baths (105°F or 40.5°C) are sometimes used in a therapeutic setting. These very hot baths, which can increase body temperature, must be used with great caution in patients with cardiac and/or circulatory problems. But a warm bath at home can also provide relief. Many people derive comfort from the whirlpool baths available in gyms or hotels. Whirlpool baths can also be installed in the home.

Joint Protection

One does not have to be a doctor to know that keeping a painful joint from moving usually lessens pain. Splints or slings successfully immobilize certain joints (shoulders, elbows, fingers, wrists, ankles, necks, and even knees). The hand splints discussed in Chapter 13 are among the most useful, as is a soft surgical collar, which reduces neck mobility. You must be careful not to use splints for too long, because they promote muscle atrophy (from disuse), reduce mobility, and can even cause osteoporosis. Some splints or braces (orthoses) allow limited joint mobility while protecting the joint from excessive stress.

Exercise

Appropriate exercise can be a good long-term method of pain relief for patients suffering from osteoarthritis. See Chapter 5 for details.

Transcutaneous Electric Nerve Stimulation (TENS)

This method involves the delivery of low-level electrical impulses over the skin of the affected area. During a typical fifteen-to-thirty-minute neuro-stimulating session, a therapist tapes electrodes to the skin near the painful joint. An electric current of variable intensity is applied; you may feel a tingling or vibrating sensation. Many patients report reduced pain from the procedure, but again it is individual. The reason for the instantaneous pain relief is unknown. Some experts speculate that the electric current releases the body's own pain-modulating chemicals (endorphins). Others believe that the electric stimulation overloads the nerve path, thereby overriding the initial pain impulse. The electrodes used in TENS are often applied to the same general areas as acupuncture points.

Massage

For her birthday Martha received a certificate for a Swedish massage. When she arrived at the spa she undressed in a dressing room, draped herself in a towel and lay on a table. Then the masseuse applied a lubricant (oil or cream) to her skin.

For a whole hour Martha relaxed while the masseuse kneaded her back, arms, legs, and shoulders. Martha never realized that she had all these different hurting muscles until the masseuse released their tension with her hands. The pushing and pinching felt relaxing and good. For a little while after the massage, the tension was gone.

There are several basic types of massage:

Effleurage: a kind of stroking during which the hand is run lightly over the skin. This type of massage is usually quite relaxing.

Petressage: compression, during which the muscles are squeezed and kneaded. Petressage mobilizes tissue fluids, stretches and breaks up soft tissue adhesions, and relaxes tense muscles.

Tapotement: percussion, or pounding of the body with the sharp edge of the hand. Tapotement stimulates nerve endings and blood circulation.

Massage is best performed by a trained person, but self-massages and even the casual kneading of a stiff, tight neck or sore shoulder dissipates pain effectively.

You may want to enhance your massage by using a menthol gel or diluted oil of wintergreen as a lubricant.

Acupuncture

The Chinese have used acupuncture for about five thousand years to remedy conditions as varied as headaches, high blood pressure, toothache, arthritis, insomnia, and nosebleeds.

According to traditional Chinese medicine, life flows along fourteen major meridians or channels, each governing a major organ, such as the heart, kidney, or stomach. Blockage of one or more meridians causes illness. Stimulation of specific acupuncture points located along the path of the meridians opens the blockage and restores equilibrium.

During treatment the acupuncturist inserts dozens of needles into acupuncture points—of which about eight hundred are known. Again, it is not clear how the technique provides pain relief, but it is believed that it reduces pain by overstimulating the surrounding nerves. It is important that the treatment be performed by a skilled acupuncturist aware of contraindications and other precautions.

Response to acupuncture is highly individual. Some people find it effective and love it, others do not.

Acupressure

Instead of acupuncture you may try acupressure. In acupressure the masseur applies gentle pressure instead of needles to the traditional acupuncture points.

Be aware that while all the above treatments may be beneficial, they may also aggravate existing symptoms. Proper supervision and careful monitoring is therefore very important.

Biofeedback

During biofeedback you train your mind to control certain body functions such as blood pressure or blood flow. Since there is a close interrelationship between pain and muscle tension, you may find it helpful to learn to relax specific muscle groups.

In one typical biofeedback setup, the patient reclines on a comfortable couch in a small, soundproof, dimly lit room. A technician tapes recording electrodes to the patient's head. These electrodes record on a special device the intensity of the muscle contraction. Additional instruments convert the muscle tension to a feedback signal, such as a click. The tenser the muscle, the faster the click. In time the patient identifies the thoughts and sensations that make the machine click faster or slower. If the training is successful, the patient gradually learns to reproduce the appropriate state of relaxation without actually being tethered to the machine. According to the National Institute of Mental Health, scientists have not quite agreed on the efficacy of biofeedback techniques.

Fatigue

Pain is tiring. So is walking about with a poorly functioning hip or knee.

To minimize your fatigue try to plan your day carefully; allow yourself plenty of time to get places or finish tasks. Do not overburden yourself, and take a rest when you feel that you are getting tired.

Ask for help. Shop from catalogues and by phone. Arrange your home and workplace so the needed equipment is close at hand. Arrange for easy transportation: taxis, cars, ambulettes. Buy gadgets designed to help you accomplish simple tasks while protecting your joints. Sources for these self-help devices are given in the *Guide to Independent Living for People with Arthritis,* which can be ordered from the Arthritis Foundation.

Sleeping

Gaby used to fall asleep as soon as her head hit her pillow, and the next morning she had a tough time getting up when the alarm went off. Now, she may fall asleep, but after a short four hours she is again wide awake. The next day her back bothers her more and she is grouchy.

Most older people have a much harder time sleeping than younger ones. Painful arthritis compounded with aging often results in marked sleeping disorders. Chronic sleep deprivation results in fatigue, increased depression, and pain.

Books and magazine articles discussing ways of overcoming sleeping problems abound. For people with painful musculoskeletal problems it may be helpful to

- have some quiet, enjoyable time before going to bed
- drink a warm, noncaffeinated beverage
- if necessary, take pain medication
- sleep on a firm mattress—neither too soft nor too hard
- keep nice and warm during the night with an electric blanket
- have a technique to go back to sleep when waking during the night (listening to music, reading, thinking of a pleasant environment)

Psychological Effects of Pain and Disability

Helen was extremely angry at her husband, but most of all at herself. She had insisted on preparing the living room for the painters. This required pushing furniture around, packing up many small objects, covering the bookcases with a sheet. Not much work, she thought. Her back "thought" otherwise. Its pain flared violently, and Helen had to take extra pain-relief medication and rest for twenty-four hours to calm it down.

David was grumpy. His friends were climbing his favorite mountain in Acadia National Park. He had to stay behind because his arthritic hip just would not let him climb over the big boulders at the foot of the trail. True, the sun was shining, the vacation was good, he was sitting on his favorite bench on the shore of a spectacular lake, reading a good book. Still, he wished he could enjoy the strenuous climb and the incredible view from the top.

Doris, too, was sad. Next Thursday was Thanksgiving. The kids were coming for dinner. She had asked her husband to buy the turkey, the cranberries, the sweet potatoes, the broccoli. Doris knew that going to the supermarket was not such a big deal, but she had always enjoyed getting the plumpest turkey, the biggest bargain. If that day's zucchini looked better than broccoli, she could rearrange her menu on the spot.

Patt looked at the full-length mirror. The silk dress looked smashing, but the clumsy sneakers ruined the whole outfit. She longed for her sleek, high-heeled pumps. Damn that knee!

Helen, David, Doris, and Patt are not angry about shopping, doing chores, sitting out an excursion, or wearing ugly sneakers. They mourn the carefree use of their bodies.

As in all grieving processes, patients afflicted by chronic disease go through certain predetermined stages: denial, anger, sadness, depression, resignation, and hopefully, making the best of what is left.

Denial

Like Helen, who insisted on pushing around the furniture, all arthritis patients know that it is difficult to come to terms with the limitations set by the disease. Yet most sufferers initially persist in habits that may increase their pain. It is important to learn to say to oneself and others: no, I can't do that.

Anger and Depression

Anger is one of the hardest emotions to cope with because it is often directed at a loved one. It is important to find ways of releasing anger appropriately so as not to damage important relationships.

It is crucial to understand the source of your anger; often it's frustration or a feeling of helplessness. It sometimes helps to exercise, keep a journal, or talk with a friend. Remember that self-help groups or telephone buddies are good substitutes for professional therapists.

Anger is often self-directed and, if allowed to smolder, may turn into depression. If it reaches that stage, you should seek the help of a specialist.

Compensation

Most patients suffering from osteoarthritis will eventually manage to come to terms with their disease. Instead of hiking up a mountain, they may take pleasure in exploring the countryside with a car. Hiring somebody else to clean the house may allow you time for other activities while retaining control of your household. Shopping from catalogues simplifies gift-giving. Take-out meals allow pain-free entertaining. Think of alternative ways to enjoy your favorite pastimes.

Mind over Matter

Self-Help Groups

Today, when there are support groups for every major disease, it is interesting to note that the first formal self-help group started in 1905. Tuberculosis was rampant then, and the treatment of choice consisted of rest cures at fancy mountain sanitariums. Not everyone could afford to go, and many had to remain in the slums of the rapidly expanding cities. It was for these patients that Dr. Joseph H. Pratt, in charge of tuberculosis patients at the Massachusetts General Hospital, organized "Classes for the Treatment of Tuberculosis in the Homes of the Poor."

The busy doctor wanted to teach his patients how to use the parks, backyards, roofs, and porches of Boston.

To Pratt's surprise the group proved that the healing and recovery rate from TB was as good as at first-class sanitaria. The pleased physician attributed the high cure rate to the interaction of the group itself, which provided each patient with a "common bond in a common disease." Pratt was impressed enough by his initial success that he devoted part of his professional career to developing self-help groups for other disorders.

Self-help groups for arthritis patients are extremely valuable. Patients share their fears and pains and exchange practical information about drugs, doctors, self-help devices, and a host of other subjects. Call the Arthritis Foundation for a self-help group meeting in your area.

A Phone Buddy, Psychotherapy

People who cannot join an Arthritis Support Group can perhaps find a phone buddy with whom to "visit" on a regular basis. Sharing common problems and solutions with someone who understands firsthand can be invaluable. Talking to a private counselor is an excellent, if expensive, alternative.

RELAXATION

Meditation

The goal of meditation is to allow the mind to relax and experience the natural silence of the inner self.

Start by making yourself comfortable, and close your eyes. Breathe deeply and regularly from your diaphragm. Feel your stomach move up and down with each deep breath.

Allow unwanted thoughts to dissolve . . . with your inner eye look at a favorite picture or a landscape. Repeat a soothing word to yourself or "listen" to the sound of the wind or the sea. Don't get upset when unbidden thoughts intrude on your consciousness, they'll go away on their own. . . .

Or try these exercises. Make yourself very comfortable and close your eyes. . . . Imagine that you are far away on a beach. . . . Feel the sun warming the skin . . . breathe in the salt air. . . . Are you going to brave the waves or are you too lazy?

Go back to the house you lived in as a teen. Open the door. Is Mom home? Is the dog wagging its tail? Where is the kitchen . . . and the bedroom? . . .

Remember . . .

Evoking a pleasant past experience is wonderfully relaxing and refreshing. It may help you to forget your pain and discomfort, for a while at least.

Almost everybody's life is so crammed full of activities that many people resent taking fifteen minutes to "do nothing." By releasing stress, time used to meditate endows you with new energy. Your increased efficiency more than compensates for the time spent meditating.

If relaxation seems to work for you, buy one of the many widely available audiocassettes. These can be obtained through catalogues, from book or record stores, or from the Arthritis Foundation.

You may also discover your own way to relax: listening to music, looking at the ocean, doing a jigsaw puzzle, or going to church.

◆ CHAPTER ◆

7

Food and Osteoarthritis

UNPROVEN REMEDIES

Rattlesnakes beware! Some faith healers believe that your dried meat is a cure-all for the pain and stiffness characteristic of arthritis. The trouble is that instead of being cured, some hopeful patients develop severe food poisoning caused by *salmonella.*

Snakes are only one of the many bizarre dietary treatments for arthritis. There are many other food-related remedies, including vinegar and honey; a white-meat-only diet; and avoidance of nightshade vegetables (tomatoes, eggplants, potatoes), sweets, or dairy products. If such dietary treatments work for you, then by all means carry on with them, although it is likely they will cause more physical and emotional harm than good.

A chronic disease like arthritis, in which pain levels rise and fall for no apparent reason, invites treatments for which there is no scientific basis. Such unproven remedies can be harmful and costly. Unfortunately, the use of these treatments may delay seeking appropriate medical care or may create a more serious problem.

In-depth investigations by leading scientists have not shown nutrition to play a major role in causing or curing arthritis. Sound nutrition, nevertheless, is an important part of your treatment plan, especially if you are overweight.

Arthritis and Body Weight

Many patients suffering from OA are overweight. Excess weight not only increases the stress on your joints, but makes it difficult to walk and carry out everyday activities.

To demonstrate to yourself the stress that weight can put on a joint, simply attach two to three pounds to your ankles and walk, or carry two five-pound packs of sugar around the block. In either case you'll note the stress. Yet many of us are ten or more pounds overweight.

Arthur B. is a typical patient with osteoarthritis. Several years ago he injured his hip in a shooting accident. The hip never healed properly, and eventually Arthur developed severe osteoarthritis of the hip. Frustrated and unhappy, Arthur gained a tremendous amount of weight, which stressed the hip and diminished even further his ability to move about—to walk, work, and enjoy life.

Arthur knew that he should exercise and lose weight, so he went to the gym to lift weights. He noticed that the guy on the bench before him lifted 240 pounds without much effort. Challenged, Arthur also selected 240-pound weights. He managed to lift them, but given his arthritis, excess weight, and the generally poor shape he was in, the effort "wiped him out." He felt discouraged and depressed.

On the way home Arthur consoled himself by eating a bacon and cheese sandwich, with ice cream for dessert. Experiencing some remorse, Arthur told himself, "Never mind that it is fattening, I'll make up for it by skipping breakfast tomorrow morning." Sore, strained muscles and depression kept Arthur from returning to the gym the next day. In fact, a week passed before he finally headed back. Arthur is an extreme case, but many patients are defeated by setting unrealistic goals for themselves.

Here are some facts about being overweight and suffering from osteoarthritis:

- Osteoarthritis affects women, with their greater tendency to be overweight, more often then men.
- Osteoarthritis affects older people who need less food (lower metabolism) and are often less active and/or have stopped exercising.
- Osteoarthritis promotes inactivity.

Unfortunately, excess weight often triggers a vicious circle:

- Excess weight stresses joints, exacerbates pain, and interferes with exercising. Extra bulk makes a person feel clumsy.
- Depression often causes overeating.
- Overeating leads to greater weight gain.

How Much Should You Weigh?

Until very recently we all believed that being thin was healthy and more attractive. This attitude was so prevalent, particularly among women, that it has given us a generation of anorexic and bulimic teenage girls. Fortunately this trend may be waning. Today we are adopting a more realistic attitude towards body weight. Moreover, it is generally accepted that body weight increases with age. Table 7-1 gives the ideal weight values recommended by the Metropolitan Life Insurance Company. Do not fret if you weigh more than the table recommends. Body weight includes both muscle tissue and fat. Athletes, for instance, may weigh more than the so-called "ideal" weight because they have well-developed muscles and little fat. Muscle tissue is heavier than fat tissue.

Diets Don't Work

Every month the cover of your favorite glossy magazine touts a new diet, such as

grapefruits for breakfast, lunch, and dinner

fifteen glasses of water a day

high-protein foods

low-protein foods

You eagerly take up the new diet and even lose a few pounds. Then you ease up on the diet. Lo and behold, before you know it, the unwanted pounds are back—with perhaps a few extra ones because your body got accustomed to using less food.

When you diet, your body uses fat reserves sparingly, responding as if you were in a famine. Unfortunately, your body keeps up the new

TABLE 7-1: *Ideal Body Weight**

Men				*Women*			
Height	Small Frame	Medium Frame	Large Frame	Height	Small Frame	Medium Frame	Large Frame
5'2"	128–134	131–141	138–150	4'10"	102–111	109–121	118–131
5'3"	130–136	133–143	140–153	4'11"	103–113	111–123	120–134
5'4"	132–138	135–145	142–156	5'0"	104–115	113–126	122–137
5'5"	134–140	137–148	144–160	5'1"	106–118	115–129	125–140
5'6"	136–142	139–151	146–164	5'2"	108–121	118–132	128–143
5'7"	138–145	142–154	149–168	5'3"	111–124	121–135	131–147
5'8"	140–148	145–157	152–172	5'4"	114–127	124–138	134–151
5'9"	142–151	148–160	155–176	5'5"	117–130	127–141	137–155
5'10"	144–154	151–163	158–180	5'6"	120–133	130–144	140–159
5'11"	146–157	154–166	161–184	5'7"	123–136	133–147	143–163
6'0"	149–160	157–170	164–188	5'8"	126–133	136–150	146–167
6'1"	152–164	160–174	168–192	5'9"	129–142	139–153	149–170
6'2"	155–168	164–178	172–197	5'10"	132–145	142–156	152–173
6'3"	158–172	167–182	176–202	5'11"	135–148	145–159	155–176
6'4"	162–176	171–187	181–207	6'0"	138–151	148–162	158–179

*Table reproduced courtesy of Metropolitan Life Insurance Company of America, 1983. Note that these weights take frame size into consideration and include shoes and indoor clothing (5 lbs for men and 3 lbs for women). The proposed weights are based on the lowest mortality rates, although body weight is only one of the many risk factors affecting life expectancy.

efficiency it learned during the diet even after normal food intake is resumed. Slower metabolism with increased food intake means overweight. This is why most everyone who diets regains the "lost" weight fast.

Long experience also has shown that diets are something people go on, and then get off. In order to lose weight permanently and keep it off, people must make lasting lifestyle changes. This can be accomplished one step at a time. The slower and smaller the changes, the more likely that people will stick with them.

Don't despair. During gradual weight loss, especially when coupled with a minimal exercise program, your body has a chance to adjust to a lower calorie intake. The weight you lose in this way will stay off.

What Is Good Nutrition?

Strictly speaking, there are no "good" or "bad" foods. Certain foods, however, should be eaten sparingly. One way of eating a healthy diet is to eat according to the food pyramid (see Figure 7-1, The Food Pyramid): morc grains, rice, beans, fruits, and vegetables; small portions of meat, fish; or poultry; and less fat. In other words, eat as your ancestors did. Foods should also be fresh and preferably cooked at home.

What Is Food Made Of?

Carbohydrates, Proteins, and Fats

Carbohydrates, proteins, and fats are *macronutrients,* meaning that the body needs these in large (macro) amounts. *Carbohydrates* and *fats* are the energy nutrients that the body burns, much as a car burns gasoline or a furnace burns oil or natural gas. The body uses carbohydrate calories more efficiently than fat calories. *Protein* is utilized to replace worn tissues and build enzymes, hormones, and other key substances that mastermind metabolism (the sum total of all the chemical transformations taking place in an organism). As a last resort, protein is burnt for energy. All food consists of protein, carbohydrates, or fat. Some foods are pure fat (oil) or pure protein (egg white) or pure carbohydrate, but most foods, especially prepared foods, are mixtures. The macronutrients are polymers like plastics, each being assembled from smaller subunits. Here are some of the major differences between the macronutrients that affect nutrition and food selection and are important enough to be listed on food labels:

Carbohydrates

There are three types of carbohydrates:

Complex carbohydrates: commonly refered to as starches (bread, rice, cereal), carbohydrates are the backbone of all diets. Starches are nutritionally valuable because they are digested slowly and thereby provide a sense of satiety. Starches are long, linked chains of glucose.

Simple or concentrated sugars: found in sweets, fruit, and vegetables. Simple sugars are digested and absorbed extremely quickly and are of limited nutritional value.

Dietary fibers: can be either soluble or insoluble. Neither type is digested, but both make an important contribution to a healthy diet. Soluble fiber, found in oat bran and certain fruits, seeds, and starchy vegetables, is believed to reduce cardiovascular risk factors. Insoluble fiber, found in whole grains, improves digestion.

Proteins

Proteins are assembled from twenty-two different amino acids. Depending on their amino acid makeup, proteins can be of high or low quality. High quality proteins are usually found in such foods as eggs, dairy products, and other foods of animal origin. Lower-quality proteins are usually of vegetable origin. Both types of protein make a crucial contribution to the diet, but those of lower quality must be carefully selected.

Fats

Fat is our most concentrated source of energy. Depending on the nature of its building blocks, it can be either saturated, monounsaturated, or polyunsaturated.

VITAMINS AND MINERALS

In addition to macronutrients, food contains minute amounts of vitamins and minerals. These are called *micronutrients.* Each micronutrient—there are about twenty in all—has a specific function. Calcium, a mineral, is used to build bones and teeth. Vitamin A is essential for vision, vitamin C maintains the health of skin and mucous membranes, and the B vitamins participate in the transformation of food into energy.

Except for calcium, micronutrients are needed in small amounts only. A well-balanced diet supplies all the necessary micronutrients. It is not easy to eat perfectly balanced meals *all* the time. To insure good nutrition, you may wish to supplement your diet with a multivitamin tablet, taken daily or three times a week. Most brand-name multivitamin tablets have the right proportion of micronutrients. Read the labels and see what fraction of the RDA (see below) is listed for each. Choose a preparation that contains about 100 percent of each micronutrient.

What Is a Good Diet?

According to the latest research, a good diet consists of approximately:

55–60 percent carbohydrates

15–20 percent protein

25–30 percent fat

Although carbohydrates and fats both supply energy, your body utilizes the carbohydrates more effectively than the twice-as-energy-dense fats. In addition to energy, starches provide vitamins, fiber, and bulk. This is especially true of enriched starches.

Dietary Goals

Eating well every day during your entire life is very important to your health. A good diet is believed to prevent or delay the onset of many chronic diseases, especially heart disease and some forms of cancer.

To help the American people to eat a healthier diet, the Surgeon General of the United States and leading scientists summarized what is meant by good nutrition in seven simple dietary goals:

- Eat a variety of foods.
- Maintain a desirable weight.
- Avoid too much fat, saturated fat, and cholesterol.
- Eat foods with adequate starch and fiber.
- Avoid too much sugar.
- Avoid too much sodium (salt).
- If you drink alcoholic beverages, do so in moderation (1 oz. 1–3 times a week).

FIGURE 7-1: *The Food Pyramid*

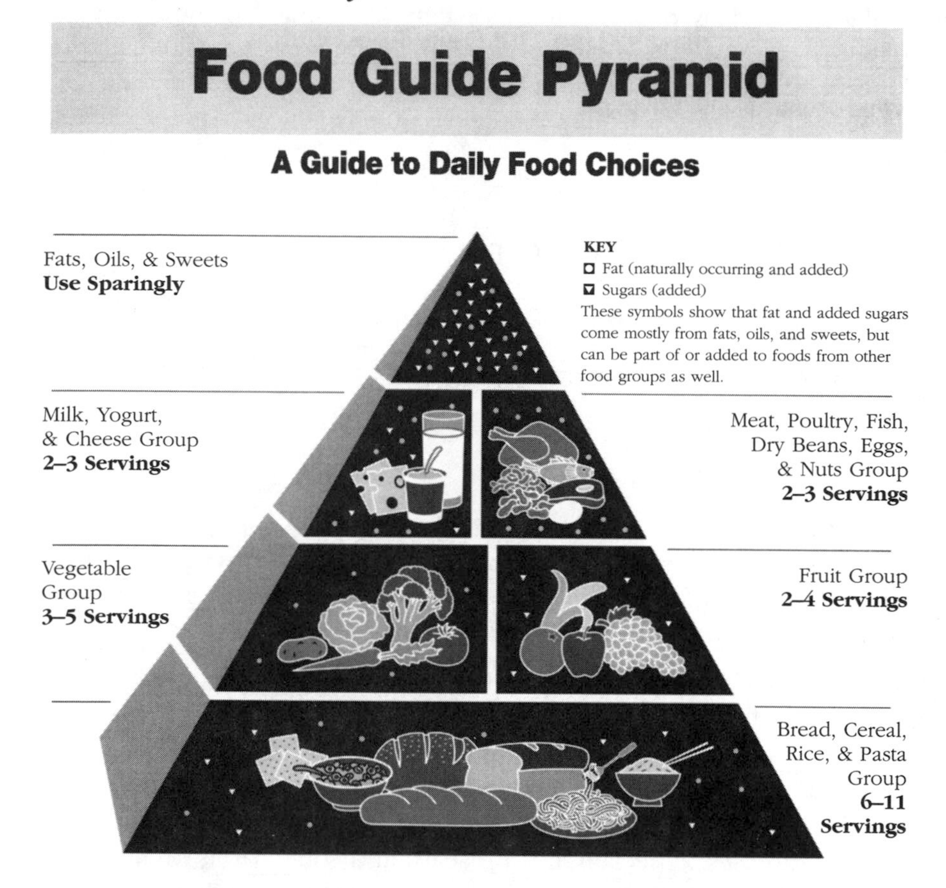

Here is a picture of the Food Pyramid. The base of the pyramid consists of food you should eat a lot of, bread, cereal, rice, and pasta (6–11 servings*/day).

The next layer up consists of fruit (2–4 servings/day) and vegetables (3–5 servings/day).

Protein foods, including meat, poultry, fish, dry beans, eggs, and nuts (2–3 servings/day) come next, and dairy foods, including milk, yogurt, and cheese (2–3 servings/day) follow. The top of the pyramid is occupied by the fats, oils, and sweets, which you should eat sparingly.

When selecting foods, always try to pick low-fat or fat-free items.

Source: U.S. Department of Agriculture/U.S. Department of Health and Human Services

*Servings, as used in these food plans, are small. You will eat 2–3 servings of bread (or meat, fat, etc.) at each meal.

The Food Pyramid

To help people nourish themselves and their families healthily, government agencies also developed systems such as the food pyramid.

CALORIES

You don't need to read this book to know that food contains calories (cal) and that consuming excess calories leads to becoming overweight. A calorie is a measure of energy. Most of the food we eat is transformed into energy for running the body. Most women require between 1,400 and 2,000 cal/day, and most men require between 1,600 and 2,400 cal/day.

STRATEGIES FOR WEIGHT LOSS

Food Diary

Most of us eat more than we think. This is why it is important to keep a simple food diary, like the one shown on page 96. Documenting what you actually eat and do can be a big eye opener.

Sometimes small changes make a big difference. For example, at breakfast you might want to use skim milk instead of whole milk, one pat of butter instead of two. Snacking on an apple instead of a doughnut would also improve the score.

There is no need to starve yourself. As a matter of fact, people who always feel hungry soon abandon their weight-loss efforts. You also don't need to give up all your favorite foods. A quick look at your food diary helps to identify favorite foods.

When you develop your meal plan, include some of these favorites. Most foods have some redeeming qualities and can be included—in moderation. Eliminating cherished foods only fosters depression. Long experience has shown that patients can lose weight without starvation or deprivation.

A Varied Diet Promotes Weight Loss

Even when you diet there is no need to be bored with meals. Variety must be built into any weight-loss program you might use. The

FIGURE 7-2: *Food Diary*

Keep an accurate record of the foods you eat. Please include the amounts of each item.

Breakfast	*Lunch*	*Dinner*	*Between Meals*	*Activity*
Sample Day				
Orange juice 4 oz. 1 c. corn flakes 1 c. whole milk 1 sl. white toast 2 pats butter 1 cup coffee 1 t. sugar	Lettuce, bacon, tomato sandwich 1/2 c. cole slaw 8 oz. diet Coke	1 chicken thigh without skin 1 baked potato 1 cup string beans 1 dinner roll 1 glass wine	1 donut 1 diet Coke	Walked 1/4 mile
Day 1				
Day 2				
Day 3				

Recording the portion size of all the foods you eat is crucial.

American Dietetic Association and organizations like Weight Watchers provide their clients with exchange lists that teach you how to "trade" one food for another. This type of system is easy to do on your own.

Take breakfast as an example. Common starch servings, such as one slice of bread, half an English muffin or bagel, one cup of cold cereal, or half a cup of hot cereal, all equal 100 calories. You can exchange one starch for another any time you like. The same exchange principle holds for lunch or dinner. A 3-ounce portion of trimmed, cooked lean meat, poultry, or fish is about 225 calories; a whole fresh fruit, a cup of fresh berries, or half a cup of canned fruit are all about 60 calories each; a cup of leafy vegetables is 25 calories; and 8 ounces of skim milk or nonfat yogurt are 80 calories. Low-calorie foods like crackers or popcorn can be eaten as snacks.

It is important that you plan your meals, select low-fat foods, and measure your portions. When you begin a weight-control program, it is helpful to plan ahead. Chart your menus for the upcoming week and stick to this food plan as well as you can. Pretty soon eating according to your food plan will become a habit.

Portion Size: The Key to Good Eating

The other important aspect of any food plan is learning how much to eat. If you eat more than your body needs, you can grow fat on pasta, or bread, or even fruit and vegetables.

Determining the serving size of the meat group is especially tricky. You may wonder how large the specified 2–3-ounce serving of cooked chicken or steak actually is. To begin with you may like to weigh the portion on a small diet scale. Another way is to measure your meat portion against your fist or the palm of your hand (minus the fingers). The sizes of both measure about a 3-ounce serving. Remember that the calories in the meat vary with its fat content.

Reading Food Labels

Today most canned and packaged foods have labels with nutrition information. These labels enable you to make good food choices; avoid excess salt, sugar, and additives; limit calories; and identify foods with high nutritional value. Though the labels provide copious information about the types of nutrients the food contains, you may only be

TABLE 7-2: *U.S. Recommended Daily Allowance (U.S. RDA) Adults and Children Over Four Years*

Protein*	65 gm*	Vitamin B-6	2.0 mg
Protein, high quality	45 gm*	Folacin	0.4 mg
Vitamin A	5,000 IU	Vitamin B-12	6 mcg
Vitamin C	60 mg	Phosphorus	1.0 gm
Thiamin	1.5 mg	Iodine	150 mcg
Riboflavin	1.7 mg	Magnesium	400 mg
Niacin	20 mg	Zinc	15 mg
Calcium	1.0	Copper	2 mg
Iron	18 mg	Biotin	0.3 mg
Vitamin D	400 IU	Pantothenic acid	10 mg
Vitamin E	30 IU		

*The recommended intake of protein in the U.S. RDA depends on the quality of the protein.

interested in part of the information, such as the number of calories per serving, the amount and type of fat or carbohydrate the food contains, or the amount of calcium or vitamins. The information on food labels is related to the Recommended Daily Allowances.

The Recommended Dietary Allowances (RDA)

In 1941 the United States Army asked the Food and Nutrition Board of the National Academy of Sciences to come up with a standard that could be used to measure the quality of the diet served to the Armed Forces. Two years later the Food and Nutrition Board published the first set of recommended daily allowances (RDA). These values, presented in table form, reflect the amount of essential nutrients that "based on the best scientific knowledge meet the known nutrient needs of practically all healthy persons." The RDAs are updated every five or more years. These small corrections reflect any newly discovered nutritional knowledge.

The complete RDA table provides information for thirty-two population groups, differing from one another with respect to age and sex. A simplified version—the U.S. RDA—is used for the nutrition facts found on food and supplement labels. Table 7-2 presents the U.S. RDA for Adults and Children Over Four Years of Age.

FIGURE 7-3: *The New Food Labels*

Nutrition Facts

Serving Size 1 cup (228g)
Servings Per Container 2

Amount Per Serving

Calories 260 Calories from Fat 120

	% Daily Value*
Total Fat 13g	**20%**
Saturated Fat 5g	**25%**
Cholesterol 30mg	**10%**
Sodium 660mg	**28%**
Total Carbohydrate 31g	**10%**
Dietary Fiber 0g	**0%**
Sugars 5g	
Protein 5g	

Vitamin A 4% • Vitamin C 2%
Calcium 15% • Iron 4%

* Percent Daily Values are based on a 2,000 calorie diet. Your daily values may be higher or lower depending on your calorie needs:

	Calories	2,000	2,500
Total Fat	Less than	100	80g
Sat Fat	Less than	20g	25g
Cholesterol	Less than	300mg	300mg
Sodium	Less than	2,400mg	2,400mg
Total Carbohydrate		300g	375g
Dietary Fiber		25g	30g

Calories per gram:
Fat 9 • Carbohydrate 4 • Protein 4

The New Food Labels

The U.S. RDA table lists daily requirements in grams (gm), milligrams (mg), micrograms (mcg), or International Units (IU). On food labels this information is converted into a percentage (%). The labels spell out the amounts in terms of the contributions that the food makes to your daily nutritional needs.

Figure 7-3 shows how the information on the labels is subdivided.

The first two sections of the label deal with serving size and calories, i.e., the amount the manufacturer considers a serving (for cereals, 1.3 oz. or 3/4 of a cup,) and the number of servings per container. All subsequent information on the package is given in terms of one serving. The next item concerns calories per serving.

The next section provides information about macronutrients: fat (nature of the fat), carbohydrate (nature of the carbohydrate), protein, cholesterol, and sodium (the latter two are believed to promote heart disease). Note that the information tells you the percentage of the daily value each of these nutrients makes towards your total dietary intake.

The next section on the label provides the same information for the micronutrients: vitamins and minerals. Note that the food shown in Figure 7-3 provides 4 percent of the U.S. RDA for vitamin A, 2 percent of the U.S. RDA for vitamin C, 15 percent of the U.S. RDA for calcium and 4 percent iron. The goal is to consume 100 percent of each nutrient daily.

The government also strictly regulates the claims a manufacturer can make for a particular food on a food label. The box on page 101 explains the meanings of key words food manufacturers are allowed to use to substantiate a specific nutritional claim.

To convince yourself how much important information you can derive from food labels, go to a supermarket and compare the labels of two cans of tuna fish, one packed in water, the other in light soybean oil. Both cans provide 100 percent of the daily protein requirement, as well as a percentage of the daily value for certain vitamins and minerals. For those interested in weight control it is important to note, however, that the number of calories provided by the tuna packed in oil is twice that of the tuna packed in water.

Exercise and Body Weight

The amount of energy your body uses every day also depends on how physically active you are. Exercise burns calories. Even light exercise burns calories. This is why it's important to record your daily exercise on the food diary.

"Burning off" food, however, is only part of the reason to exercise. Exercise maintains good muscle tone and thereby helps patients remain fit in spite of arthritis. (For details see Chapter 5.)

Common Key Words Used on Food Labels

Fat free: The food must contain less that 0.5 gram of fat per serving.

Low Fat: Only 3 grams of fat (or less) per serving.

Lean: The food must contain less than 10 grams of fat, 4 grams of saturated fat, and 95 milligrams of cholesterol per serving.

Light (Lite): The food must contain either one half fewer calories or no more that half the fat of the higher-calorie version, or no more that half the sodium of the regular version.

Cholesterol Free: Less than 2 milligrams of cholesterol and no more than two grams of saturated fat per serving.

Tips on How to Lose Weight (Behavior Modification)

Losing weight and keeping it off usually involves a permanent alteration in eating behavior. Such behavior modification is now used to help people change ingrained habits in many aspects of life. Here are behavior modification suggestions related to eating.

- Lose weight very slowly—a quarter or a half pound a week will do.
- Develop a reasonable, flexible eating plan and stick with it.
- Do not weigh yourself every day. Instead, ask yourself whether your clothes fit better or whether you can move more easily.
- Set yourself small goals. If you love ice cream, have it once or twice a week instead of every day.
- Try new, lower-calorie foods. Substitute baked potatoes for french fries or baked sliced potatoes for potato chips.
- Read food labels. They tell you how many calories a portion of food contains and how much carbohydrate, protein, and fat (see above).

- Eat meals and snacks at the same time each day, and decide beforehand what you are going to eat. You may also wish to measure the amount of food you will eat. Do not skip meals, because then you will eat more at the next meal. Stop eating when you are full. Plan and limit your snacks.
- Eat slowly, savor each bite, and pause between them. Concentrate on your meal; do not let anything distract you.
- Shop carefully: planning helps eliminate overstocked cabinets. Always shop from a prepared shopping list and never shop when you are hungry.
- Always read food labels of unfamiliar foods. Select water-packed tuna, unsweetened fruit, ice milk, low-fat dairy products, unsweetened cereals. Avoid the food aisles that stock your "trigger" foods.
- Cook only small amounts of food. Do not nibble on food while cooking. Once you are ready to eat, measure your food portions and don't have seconds. Modify or avoid recipes that require a lot of calorie-dense ingredients.
- Set yourself reasonable goals, such as the following:
    - I will not have butter on my roll the next time I go to a restaurant.
    - I will buy a bagel or an apple at the coffee cart instead of a doughnut.
    - I will use lemon instead of dressing on my salad; I will not use sugar in my coffee.
    - Next time I feel like eating, I will call a friend.
    - I will exercise three minutes on the treadmill today, four minutes tomorrow.
    - I will order a baked potato instead of French fries.
- Celebrate accomplishments with a reward like buying a magazine, a book, flowers, a piece of clothing, or going to the movies. Don't reward yourself with food.
- Buy lunch at a salad bar or bring prepared food from home. This is cheap and easy.

- Never arrive at a party famished. We all eat more when hungry. During the cocktail hour or at a buffet, taste everything, but concentrate on low-calorie foods such as celery and carrot sticks. Keep your hands busy with diet soda, club soda, or juice. Avoid chips, dips, nuts, and other snacks that invite compulsive consumption. Limit yourself to mineral water, low-calorie sodas or bloody Mary mix. Sip slowly. If you must drink, have one serving of light beer, wine, or hard liquor without sugar-laden mixers. Concentrate on conversation.

Cooking in Spite of Arthritis

Some people love to cook, others hate it. Whether you like it or not, cooking and cleaning up may be difficult because of fatigue, hands rendered clumsy by arthritis, and painful weight-bearing joints. As always, determination and inventiveness will triumph over physical limitation. Chapters 13 and 14 of *The Guide to Independent Living for People with Arthritis,* published by the Arthritis Foundation, discusses kitchen planning and meal preparation in great detail.

Here are a few overall suggestions:

- Use laborsaving devices (mixers, blenders, electric can openers).
- Plan meals ahead of time and assemble everything you need before you start to cook.
- Slide heavy pots instead of carrying them.
- Use cut-up vegetables from a salad bar or the vegetable section of the supermarket.
- Sit while you work.
- Keep dish washing to a minimum by using disposable pans or cooking in a microwave oven.
- Cook extra food and freeze extra single-size portions for later use.
- Find a grocery store that takes phone orders and delivers. Select a store that carries a wide variety of vegetables, fruit, and low-calorie packaged foods.

◆ PART ◆

II

Surgical Management of Osteoarthritis

◆ CHAPTER ◆

8

Should You Have Surgery?

Claire B.'s right knee hurt; not at night, not while she walked around the house, but whenever she went shopping, took a walk, or played with her grandchildren. Her X ray showed that the cartilage in the knee joint was completely worn away, and that bone rubbed on bone. But each time she asked her surgeon for a new knee, he told her to wait.

Bert E.'s hip was shot. He could no longer play tennis or hike up a mountain. For a while the pain was so severe that he could not sleep at night. His doctor said that medically he was ready to have a new hip, but that it was his decision. "You tell us when you want your hip," the doctor concluded. Bert, however, is afraid of this extensive operation.

"I have high blood pressure and am overweight. Who knows what I'll be like after such major surgery. I manage all right. The new pain medication my doctor prescribed helps. I have handicapped license plates on my car, drive myself everywhere, and park near where I want to be. I stay behind when my family goes hiking. A new hip might enable me to play tennis and to travel more extensively. Someday maybe, but not now."

Surgery intended to reconstruct joints destroyed by arthritis usually is elective, which means that it is not absolutely necessary to preserve life.

Nevertheless, choosing not to have the surgery may not be your most cautious choice. In many instances, repairing one arthritic joint can prevent another one from being overstressed. Total joint replacement almost always alleviates pain. It enables you to be more active physically, thereby promoting fitness, weight control, and cardiovascular health. Surgery of the hands improves function and appearance.

Any surgery, however, is risky, time-consuming, and expensive. Certain types of joint surgery require lengthy rehabilitation. This chapter reviews factors that you must take into consideration before you plan to undergo joint surgery.

Factors to Consider

Before deciding for or against surgery, evaluate the following factors:

Pain: Pain relief is the most immediate and dramatic result of joint replacement surgery. Assess your pain. How bad is it? Does it keep you from sleeping? Does it keep you from enjoying life? Can it no longer be controlled by medication? Does the pain depress you?

Lifestyle: How much does your arthritic joint interfere with work and play? Can you no longer do the things you need or want to do? Ask your doctor what the surgery will do for you.

Extent of Your Arthritis: Is your discomfort caused mostly by one diseased joint or by several? If several joints are involved, discuss with your physician which is the most important to replace first. For instance, hip or knee replacement requires serviceable shoulders and elbows so that you can use crutches.

Other Diseases: Take into account other health factors that might be affected by surgery. For example: Will the physiological stress of the operation overstrain your ailing heart? Or will improved physical function enable you to exercise more and improve your cardiovascular fitness? Similar considerations apply to other chronic ailments like diabetes or kidney disease.

Time Commitment: Total joint replacement and its rehabilitation time can take anywhere from two to four months. Consider whether you can easily take such a large slice of time out of your life.

Cost of Surgery: Total joint replacement is an expensive procedure. Find out whether your insurance (Medicare, Medicaid, or private) pays for the operation. Remember that anesthesia often involves a separate bill.

Rehabilitation: Discuss with your doctor the length and nature of the postsurgical rehabilitation. Ask whether you will require crutches? A walker? Splints? Special rehabilitation exercises? Evaluate your ability to follow such a treatment plan. Will you be able to follow this rigorous routine at home?

Risk Taking: Are you willing to put up with the potential complications that may result from the surgery?

Talking to Another Patient: To help you decide, ask your doctor for the name and telephone number of one or more patients who has had a similar operation. You will learn a lot from their experiences.

Getting a Second Opinion: Today most insurance companies require a second opinion before they agree to pay for surgery. Your physician will welcome your getting a second opinion. Do not be afraid to ask him or her for the name of a consultant. Keep in mind that this second doctor is not necessarily more knowledgeable or correct than the first doctor. If need be, you can even consult a third doctor.

Types of Surgery

During the past two decades the types of surgical interventions used to correct arthritic deformities have undergone a dramatic change. Currently, total joint replacement is the treatment most often used for hips, knees, and shoulders requiring surgery because of osteoarthritic damage. The success rate is so high that other surgical modalities, including osteotomy and arthrodesis, are seldom used. Less extensive surgery can often be performed by arthroscopy.

Arthroscopy

An arthroscope is a small, pencil-sized fiber-optic instrument used for both diagnosis and surgery. For diagnosis the instrument is connected to a small camera viewer the physician uses to examine the inside of the joint and assess the exact nature of the damage.

The arthroscope is used to remove floating pieces of cartilage and bone fragments from the joint cavity. This osteoarthritic debris often interferes with pain-free joint movement.

Initially, arthroscopes were mostly used to address knee problems. Today they are used increasingly for shoulders and, to a lesser degree, elbows and ankles. They are particularly beneficial in the treatment of sports injuries. However, arthroscopic surgery is not entirely risk-free.

Complications may include infection and/or residual pain and stiffness. (For details, see Chapter 10, "The Knee".)

Osteotomy

"*Tom*" is Greek for cutting, and osteotomy means "cutting of the bone." During an osteotomy procedure the surgeon may remove or add a wedge of bone, thereby realigning a joint and restoring its pain-free function. The aim of an osteotomy is to shift weight-bearing from one part of the joint to another. The advantage of the procedure is that it does not use any foreign parts in the joint. Unfortunately, it's not easy to predict how much pain relief might be achieved by the surgery. Moreover, arthrodesis may make a subsequent total joint replacement more difficult. The procedure is mostly used for hips and knees for younger patients who might overstress a man-made prosthesis or "outlive" one or two implants.

Arthrodesis

Arthrodesis refers to the fusion of the two or more bones in a joint. The procedure eliminates pain and provides stability. The operation is quite debilitating, since a fused joint loses its function. In the past, arthrodesis was used for both hips and knees. Today arthrodesis is mostly used for highly unstable wrists or failed, infected knee replacements. The operation is sometimes used for patients who are too young or too active to have a total hip replacement.

Total Joint Replacement (Arthroplasty)

Today total joint replacement is the most commonly used surgical procedure for patients with advanced osteoarthritis. Although many joints can be replaced (see Figure 8-1), hip and knee replacements are by far most common, exceeding 300,000 operations annually.

The advent of total joint replacement is the most glorious chapter in orthopedic arthritis surgery during the twentieth century. When indicated, it is a miraculous cure for those who would otherwise be crippled or wheelchair-bound by arthritis.

Joint replacement as we know it today dates from the 1960s, when Sir John Charnley, M.D., developed a functional hip in a rather unknown hospital in Wrightington, England.

FIGURE 8-1: *Joints That Can Be Reconstructed Surgically*

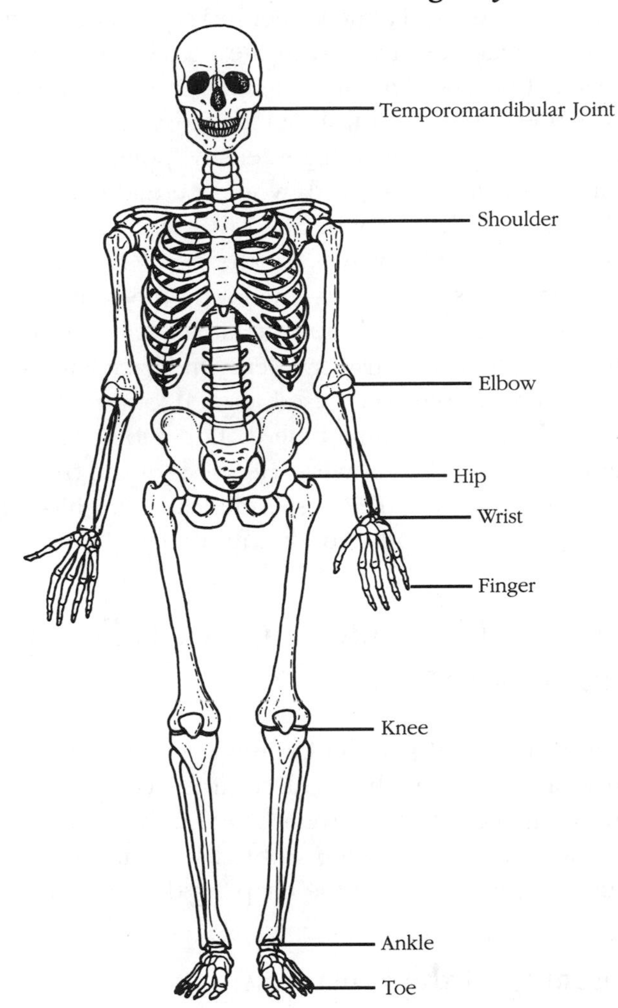

Success with the hip encouraged surgeons to replace other joints. Figure 8-1 shows joints that can now be replaced. The replacement of most of these joints is detailed in subsequent chapters.

The hip is a ball-and-socket joint (see Figure 9-1). Its shape makes it extremely stable. Because it is such an important, centrally located joint, its destruction by arthritis is particularly disabling. For decades surgeons repaired arthritic hips with metal-only components. One common operation was the insertion of a metal cup into the acetabulum portion of the pelvis. Metal hinges, fastened to bone with screws or wires, were used to fix knees. Neither repair lasted very long. The non-anchored metal cup inserted in the acetabulum shifted; the wires and screws that fastened the hinged-knee prosthesis loosened.

Charnley conceived fashioning one side of the joint out of metal and the other half of a high-density polymer (plastic). The metal-polymer interface, he figured, would permit low-friction motion.

For the hip, Charnley decided to use metal to replace the head of the femur. He used polymer for the cup. One of the major problems confronting the surgeon was anchoring the prosthesis to the skeleton. Dentistry, which used cement to attach crowns to teeth in the wet mouth, supplied the answer. Methylmethacrylate cement, which sets quickly, is now commonly used in total joint replacement.

It took Charnley some time to find a biocompatible polymer that would withstand years of wear. He tried several before settling on high-density polyethylene. The first American total hip replacements were performed in New York City during the late 1960s.

Possible Complications of Total Joint Replacement

Unfortunately, total joint replacement is not a panacea. Complications arise in a few cases. The most common complications are loosening, dislocation, and infection. Wear of the polyethylene is also looming as a long-term problem. Here is a brief look at the major complications, discussed more closely in the chapters dealing with individual joints.

Loosening of the Prosthesis:

As prostheses age, even the best, most successfully implanted ones have a tendency to loosen. The time at which this occurs is unpredictable. Three factors seem to play a major role:

- the skill of the surgeon
- the mechanical stress to which the implant is subjected (body weight and activity)
- biological factors related to bone loss surrounding the implant; this itself may be related to the wear of the plastic

To keep complications to a minimum

- select a competent surgeon
- keep your body weight within reasonable limits (see Chapter 7)
- delay surgery until you are less active

Infection

Infection of an artificial joint is a very serious complication that occurs in about half a percent of all cases. To minimize the risk of an infectious organism entering the wound, the surgery is performed in as sterile an environment as possible. A general airflow system, ultraviolet light, and "spacesuits" are used during surgery to keep bacterial contamination to a minimum.

Prophylactic antibiotics, administered prior to surgery and for one or two days thereafter, help minimize infections related to the surgery. To reduce the risk of postsurgical infections

- have your teeth repaired prior to joint surgery
- treat existing infections, such as those of the genitourinary tract and the skin
- take prophylactic antibiotics before dental procedures (including visits to the dental hygienist) and prior to invasive diagnostic tests
- inform new physicians and dentists that you have an artificial joint

Preparing for Surgery

Selecting the Hospital

The success of your surgery depends not only on the skill of your surgeon, but also on the staff members of the hospital who provide general care, physical therapy, and occupational therapy. It is also important that the hospital's staff members can provide special care if complications develop. It is best to select a hospital that not only has excellent orthopedists, therapists, or rheumatologists, but also highly qualified cardiologists and infectious-disease specialists.

On the other hand, you may wish to have your surgery close to home. In either case, visit the hospital(s) you contemplate going to. Is the staff friendly? Does the hospital have an adequate physical therapy department with modern equipment? Talk to someone who used this hospital and get his or her opinion.

In the end, however, you may not have a choice, since your doctor(s) may not be able to practice at your first-choice hospital.

Medical Evaluation

Once you have decided to have the surgery, you should

- have a *complete medical examination* by your personal internist, with special emphasis on evaluation of heart, lung, and kidney function, as well as circulatory or neurological problems (infections of any kind—skin, urinary tract, gynecologic—must be identified and treated)
- *visit your dentist* (again, have all existing or potential sources of infections identified and treated)

Nonmedical Preparations

Surgery is emotionally taxing and physically debilitating. Here are some tips on how to reduce overall stress before, during, and after the operation.

Insurance: Examine your health insurance contract to see whether the following are covered:

physical therapy (at home and in the hospital)

private duty nursing

assistive devices (crutches, toilet seat, etc.)

home health care

disability

If you have any questions call your insurance company. Write down the name of the person you spoke with.

Health Care Proxy, Advanced Directives: Unless you have done so already, appoint a health care proxy who can make appropriate decisions should you be unable to do so.

Other Money Matters: Do as much paperwork as possible beforehand. Arrange to pay your rent, credit card, and telephone bills before you enter the hospital, and "fatten up" your checking account if you can.

Help: Hospital stays and major surgery are exhausting. When you come home, you will be tired and handicapped. Arrange to have somebody stay with you during the first week(s). Arrange for someone to care for your plants and pet(s) during and after your hospital stay.

Home Rearrangement: Rearrange your home so that you can live in it comfortably with your crutches, cane, walker or nonfunctional hands. Check for the following:

- **Bathroom:** Is it easy to maneuver in? If you had hip surgery you will need a raised toilet seat. Do you have a stall shower? If not, you may need to find an alternative if you cannot climb into the tub.
- **Sitting:** Sitting on a high chair (hips higher than knees) is essential after hip surgery. Many hospitals have special high chairs for their freshly operated patients and it is nice to have such a chair when you come home. If possible, buy, borrow, or rent such a chair before you go to the hospital.
- **Kitchen and Eating:** After surgery you may have trouble shopping and cooking. Before surgery, prepare and freeze your own home-cooked meals. Stock up on staples and frozen dinners. Arrange for Meals on Wheels to deliver food.
- **Bedroom:** If you live in a two-floor house, you may prefer sleeping downstairs until you can manage the stairs easily.
- **Activities:** Stock up on books, handicrafts, videotapes, jigsaw puzzles, and other hobbies you're usually too busy to enjoy.

More About Surgery

Anesthesia

The discovery in 1799 that nitrous oxide (laughing gas) temporarily eliminates pain was essential to the development of surgery. The early anesthetics were gases which, when inhaled, curtailed the transmission of sensations (including pain) through the nerves to the brain.

Preoperative Checklist

Discuss with Doctor: How long surgery will last; type of anesthesia that will be used; medications; autologous blood donation.

Schedule Appointments With: Your internist, dentist, and mental health counselor.

Packing for the Hospital: Take as little as possible. The hospital will supply you with gowns, toiletries and a television set. Leave valuables at home. Items you may need or want include: slippers, toothbrush, toothpaste, bathrobe, and glasses.

Also Take: An inexpensive watch. A radio or some favorite tapes. Light reading matter. Old magazines. Knitting or needlework. Phone numbers, stationery, and stamps.

Anesthesia usually causes temporary loss of memory. You will have no recollection of the surgery or of the pain that accompanied it. Today anesthesiology is a major medical specialty.

Your anesthesiologist will probably see you before the surgery and explain the type of anesthesia to be used. He or she will be present during the entire operation, administering the anesthetic and monitoring your respiration, blood pressure, and other vital signs. During the operation the anesthesiologist adjusts the amount of anesthetic administered so that it lasts as long as necessary, but no longer.

Most of us are familiar with anesthesia. Even if you have never had surgery, you have probably had a local anesthetic during dental work. Many patients, nevertheless, are scared of anesthesia, fearing that they will not wake up or that its effects will be lasting.

As always, the best antidote to fear is understanding how a procedure works. Anesthetics are narcotic drugs that induce sleep. They vary in their length of action. The effect of some is very short (minutes), while others last much longer (hours). You would probably have a short-acting anesthetic during a tooth extraction and a long one during joint replacement.

Three types of anesthesia are used for total joint replacements: general, spinal, and nerve block. In general, physicians prefer to administer the smallest amount of anesthetic that will do the trick. Therefore, local (regional or nerve block) anesthesia is usually preferred to general anesthesia.

No matter which type of anesthesia is selected, the anesthesiologist first will administer a dose of a milder, sleep-inducing medication. You will become very drowsy.

General anesthesia: This is administered through a breathing tube attached to a respirator that also delivers oxygen. A short-acting general anesthetic (pentothal or other) is injected so you do not feel the breathing tube being inserted into your trachea. During the surgery the respirator will do your breathing.

Spinal anesthesia: The spinal canal houses the major nerve paths that transmit sensation from all parts of the body to the brain. When an anesthetic is injected into the spinal canal, it temporarily interrupts nerve impulse transmission. In principle, patients under spinal anesthesia are aware of their surroundings. In practice, however, patients are in a drug-induced twilight sleep and don't remember anything.

Nerve blocks (regional anesthesia): Nerve blocks are used mainly for hand and foot surgery. In these cases the anesthetic is injected near the group of nerves that supply the particular limb.

Be sure to discuss your anesthesia with your physician during your preadmission visit. Ask whether it will be general, spinal, or regional. Discuss any misgivings you may have.

Blood Transfusion

In the beginning of the current medical revolution, blood banks harvested blood from anyone willing to donate it. But in light of the increased risks of hepatitis and AIDS contaminations, blood donation centers have tightened their testing procedures. Today the American blood supply is safe, with a vanishingly small risk of contamination.

Nevertheless, these fears have spurred the concept of autologous blood transfusions—where you supply your own blood if you know that you are likely to require blood during a planned operation. The blood will then be reinfused when needed.

The National Blood Resource Center of the National Institutes of Health suggests the following guidelines for autologous blood donors:

- Patients can donate blood when they know that they will have surgery in two or more weeks.

- Patients should find out whether, and how much, blood may be required during or after surgery. Two to three pints are usual for a total hip or knee.
- Age is not much of a limiting factor. Provided they are in good health, many elderly patients can donate their own blood as readily as younger ones can. Blood has been collected from children as young as eight years of age.

Patients planning to undergo orthopedic surgery are ideal candidates for autologous blood transfusion. In general, they are healthy, and their surgery is planned, rather than an emergency. Total joint replacement operations are often associated with considerable blood loss, and postsurgical blood transfusions speed recovery.

A healthy body manufactures new blood very quickly. To prevent possible iron depletion, your doctor may advise you to take iron pills (300 mg three times a day is usual) for several weeks before the blood donation. On the day of your blood donation, eat a good breakfast. You can have lunch if your appointment is in the afternoon. Avoid eating fatty foods.

The blood donation itself usually takes between five and twenty minutes. There are no major risks in donating blood. One pint of blood is collected during each donation.

Depending on the number of pints of blood you may require during surgery, you should begin planning your autologous blood donations four to six weeks prior to your surgery. Unless absolutely essential, no blood should be collected during the seventy-two hours before the actual surgery.

Medication

Discuss, with your physician, all the medications that you are taking (both prescription and over-the-counter), and ask whether you should continue taking them before the operation and during your stay in the hospital. Aspirin, for example, affects blood coagulation and must be discontinued three weeks prior to surgery.

In the hospital, do not take any medication on your own, but make sure that hospital attendants (physicians, nurses, etc.) are aware of your needs.

If you are able to, examine the medications you are given in the hospital. Ask what the pills are for. If applicable, ask why

certain medications that you take regularly (blood pressure medication, heart medication, diuretics) are omitted.

Be aware that surgery may alter the dosage (amount) of certain medications that you require. The stress of the surgery often increases the need for insulin, oral antidiabetics, or corticosteroids and decreases the need for antihypertensive medication.

YOUR HOSPITAL STAY

Same-Day Surgery

Because of escalating hospital costs, many surgical procedures are now done on the day the patient checks into the hospital. Patients arrive in a special same-day surgery suite at the hospital the morning or afternoon of the surgery and wake up in their room after it is all over.

Both patients and hospital staff agree that admitting surgery patients the day before the procedure was nicer and neater. It allowed patients time to get settled and adjust for the next day. Today, most insurance companies simply won't pay for this extra presurgical day, so most hospitals have an outpatient preadmission system.

As with other aspects of medicine, same-day admission places greater responsibility on you, the patient. For example, you are responsible for not eating after midnight and omitting breakfast. Any type of food or drink increases the likelihood of aspiration (reflux of acid stomach content into the respiratory tract) during anesthesia and surgery.

Preadmission testing, done in addition to the in-depth evaluation by your own doctor, is extensive and thorough. The preadmission procedure may take place a few days before your actual surgery in a specially equipped area of the hospital. You will progress from one health professional to the next, checking in with nurses, ECG technicians, phlebotomists who take blood samples, operating-room schedulers, hospital-room assigners, clerical workers, and financial prescreeners.

You will leave the admissions office with a folder explaining the hospital rules and regulations as well as information pertaining to your rights and regulations (see Appendix II). If everything is satisfactory, you can go home.

The Operating Room

The operating room is discussed extensively in conjunction with the surgery of specific joints (see Chapters 9 through 14). After the operation is completed, all patients go to the recovery room. Be sure to tell the doctor whom to call after the operation is completed.

The Recovery Room

Here physicians and nurses continue to monitor vital signs as the anesthesia wears off. You may still not be awake because of the prolonged effect of the sleep-inducing medication. When stable, you are transferred to your own hospital room.

When you awake you may feel disoriented. There will be pain, but it will be different than before the surgery. It will take a few days before the major discomforts of extensive surgery disappear: the myriad tubes that drain away your urine and the fluid produced by your wound and the intravenous lines that deliver antibiotics and glucose.

You are mistaken, however, if you think that you can just lie back and suffer. Physical therapists come and move your joints, doing passive exercises. The nurse may ask you to blow into a bottle to clear your lungs.

Private Duty Nursing

Hospital nurses are chronically overworked. Many patients, even those of moderate means, feel that it is helpful, even essential, to have a private duty nurse or aide during the initial day or days after surgery. These nurses will always be there to adjust the pillows, raise or lower the bed, reposition your limb, bring the bedpan, help you get out of bed, check on whether you can have extra pain medication, or bring you water. In short, it is their job to make you more comfortable. Some patients hire an extra nurse just for the night.

Many insurance companies provide for a limited number of days of private duty nursing. You can hire a registered nurse (RN), a practical nurse, or a nursing aide. The RNs are most expensive, and the aides cost the least. Orthopedic patients, whose needs during recovery are more for comfort than medical care, may do very well with an aide.

Physical Therapy

Very soon you are ready to get out of bed. That's when rehabilitation begins. A physical therapist or nurse will help you get up the first time. Always sit up slowly, and dangle your feet before standing up. You have undergone major surgery, and it takes time for your blood circulation to adjust.

You may have to relearn to walk. It may be painful. At first you will use a walker, but as soon as you have mastered that you will be switched to crutches. Given hospital costs, you will be discharged from the hospital as soon as you can manage on your own.

Discharge, however, does not mean the end of your physical therapy. The physical rehabilitation of the joint is by far the most important aspect of your recovery. Often you can perform the simple exercises you were taught at the hospital on your own, at home. I know one total hip patient who spent twenty minutes each day marching around his dining room table.

Other patients, especially those with new knees or shoulders, require exercises performed and/or supervised by a physical therapist. Arrange for home visits or for transportation to take you to the physical therapist.

Occupational Therapy

You will be sent home long before you can do everything. An occupational therapist will teach you how to protect your new joint and how to relearn basic skills. (For more details, see chapters dealing with specific joints, especially Chapter 13, "The Hand, Wrist, and Elbow.")

Going Home

If you have hip or knee surgery, or if you have to climb many stairs to get to your apartment, you may want an ambulette to take you home from the hospital. Doctors as well as insurance companies differ on this issue, so check with your doctor and hospital social worker a few days before discharge. Otherwise a relative or friend can pick you up by car or taxi. The trip home will exhaust you, so go straight to bed when you get there.

THE POSTSURGICAL VISIT

The postsurgical visit is usually scheduled four to six weeks after surgery, unless you need to come in sooner to have stitches removed. It is often a very upbeat visit. Your joint should be less painful and, by now, halfway functional. The new joint is x-rayed, and hopefully looks perfect. You are on your way to a perfect recovery.

◆ CHAPTER ◆

9

The Hip

The hip joint is deeply hidden within the pelvic cavity, yet its importance was not lost upon our ancestors. The Bible records that when Samson, Israel's legendary strongman, freed his country from the Philistines, "he smote (his enemies mercilessly) hip and thigh." Today we use *hip* to cheer, as in "hip, hip, hurray," and someone who is aware of the latest trends is said to be "hip."

No one affected by advanced osteoarthritis of the hip thinks kindly of this centrally located joint, which often renders life totally unbearable. Consequently, in orthopedics no surgical achievement will ever equal the excitement of the successful replacement of a diseased or broken hip by a new functional one. Before the advent of the total hip replacement, dysfunctional hips were a major cause of disability, condemning thousands of patients to sit in wheelchairs or walk on crutches. Today about 110,000–120,000 hips are replaced annually in the United States alone, with good to excellent outcome in 95 percent of the patients.

Anatomy of the Hip

Bony Structure

The hip joint, unlike the knee, elbow, or shoulder, cannot easily be felt. A ball-and-socket joint, it is located about four inches deep in the groin.

FIGURE 9-1: *The Hip: Bony Structure*

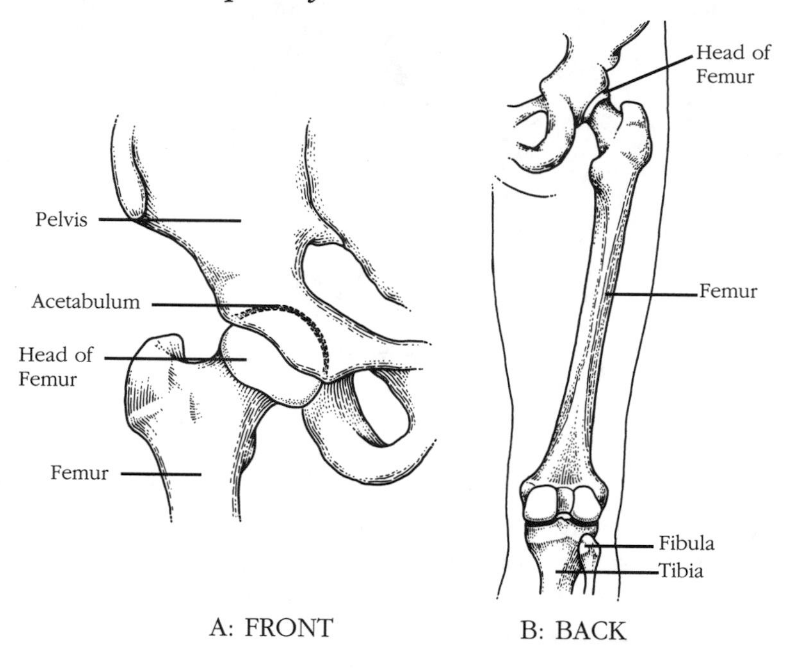

A. The hip is a ball-and-socket joint. The ball part is the head of the femur or thigh bone, and the socket is the acetabulum part of the pelvic bone. Because the acetabulum is deep, the hip joint is extremely stable. The hip joint is kept in place by a dense, fibrous capsule and numerous ligaments. **B.** Shows the relationship of the hip to the knee as seen from the back.

The ball part is the head of the femur or thigh bone, and the socket is the *pelvic bone* or *acetabulum,* from the Latin for "vinegar cup."

The hip joint connects the *femur* with the pelvis. The femur is the longest bone of the body. The lower end of the femur terminates in the knee. At its upper end the femur divides into the *greater trochanter* of the femur and the *femoral neck* which terminates in the *femoral head.* The femoral head is two thirds of an almost perfect sphere. There is a very close fit between the head of the femur and the acetabulum located on the outer side of the pelvis. The acetabulum itself is a rather deep cup enclosing 40 percent of the head of the femur. Contact is increased to 50 percent by a layer of extremely dense tissue (labrum, or lip) that protrudes on both sides of the acetabulum. In healthy persons the surfaces of the hip joint are smooth and five to eight times more slippery than ice.

The entire hip joint is enclosed in a dense, fibrous capsule that is lined by the synovium. The capsule is reinforced by numerous ligaments. As usual, the synovium secretes small amounts of lubricating fluid.

Soft Tissues

Muscles

A large joint like the hip requires large muscles. Three of the principal muscle groups of the hip are the *flexors* (e.g., the *iliopsoas* muscle), the *extensors* (e.g., the *gluteus maximus*), and the *abductors* (e.g., the *gluteus medius*). The first permit the hip to bend, the second straighten it, the third keep the pelvis from dipping (lurching) when you walk. The gluteus maximus is what gives the buttocks their bulk. Several other muscles, including the abductors and rotators, enable the hip and leg to perform other movements such as rotating and moving in and out. The muscles and ligaments of the hip are cushioned by numerous small bursae.

Nerves

The three principal nerves transmitting messages about the hip are the *sciatic nerve,* the *femoral nerve,* and the *obturator nerve.* The sciatic nerve is the largest nerve of the body. It runs from the lumbar region of the spine, down the pelvis, to the buttocks and the back of the leg. The femoral nerve also starts in the lumbar region but runs down the front of the thigh. The obturator nerve runs from the groin down the inner part of the thigh.

Stability

The rounded femoral head, which fits so well into the deep acetabulum, and the strong ligaments and muscles that surround the joint contribute to the stability of the hip joint. It usually takes a major impact, such as a car accident, to dislocate a normal hip. On the other hand, some people are born with a dislocated hip, which, even when treated, can result in osteoarthritis in early adulthood.

Osteoarthritis of the Hip

Diagnosis

Pain is usually the first symptom of osteoarthritis of the hip. During the initial consultation a doctor evaluates the pain, function, and mobility of the hip and orders X rays.

Pain

The pain in any joint can originate in that joint or can be referred from elsewhere in the body. In the case of the hip, the pain may originate in the spine, the groin, the sacroiliac joint, or even the abdomen. Orthopedic surgeons always carefully evaluate the joints adjacent to the one that hurts, because all these may use the same pain pathway. Pain in the hip often originates in the back. One way of distinguishing pain originating in the hip from referred pain is that true hip pain is always aggravated by walking but referred back pain is not automatically so. Pain originating in the back is often aggravated during prolonged sitting.

Once the doctor establishes the source of your pain, he or she will carefully evaluate the intensity and duration of the pain during routine activities. Does the pain follow strenuous exertions, such as walking or lifting heavy objects? Pain perception is highly individualized, and patients are often asked to evaluate their pain on a scale of 1 to 10.

Function

The function of the hip can be impaired by pain, muscle weakness, muscle spasms, or restricted mobility of the joint. During evaluation patients are asked to walk, bend, and stretch. Typically an osteoarthritic hip often causes a limp that becomes especially marked later in the day and makes stair climbing difficult. Doctors usually ask their patients about the distance (e.g., the number of city blocks) they can walk comfortably.

Range of Motion

A physical examination indicates varying degrees of impairment of the hip's range of motion. A healthy hip flexes (bends), extends (straightens), rotates inward (internal rotation), and rotates outward (external rotation). With osteoarthritis the internal rotation is often affected first, then the external rotation, and then, finally, extension and flexion. As the osteoarthritis of the hip increases, everyday activities—such as sitting, tying shoelaces, and cutting toenails—and even sexual function become difficult.

How Osteoarthritis Affects the Hip

Mild Osteoarthritis

The hip joints of all older persons show some wear and tear, but fortunately most people do not develop clinically significant osteoarthritis of the hip. Most often, mild osteoarthritis of the hip responds to medical management, including NSAIDs, rest, and exercise. As stressed previously, the pain experienced by the patient is not necessarily related to the extent of the osteoarthritis. Depending on its location, a small area of degeneration may be more debilitating and painful than a large one. Much depends also on the pain tolerance of the patient and his or her activity level.

Scientists attribute the initial pain of an osteoarthritic hip to a minor disintegration of the cartilage of the hip. The resulting debris may cause local inflammation. The osteoarthritic changes at this stage are very localized or, as doctors say, "focal." At this stage, there may not be any X-ray changes. As the disease progresses, more cartilage is lost and small bone spurs form at the periphery of the joint.

As always, the body attempts to minimize pain, which, in the case of joints, translates into loss of motion and function. Such protection always results in loss of muscle strength.

Moderate Osteoarthritis

Gradually, as the disease progresses, cartilage rubs away. The body may respond by forming bone spurs. The resulting osteophytes not only interfere with the smooth function of the joint but also destroy the exquisitely engineered shape of the hip joint. All these changes cause the space between the femoral head and the acetabulum to narrow. The disease spreads and eventually involves the entire joint. The major symptom is pain, which gradually becomes more severe. There is also decreased rotation of the entire joint, although flexion (bending) and extension (straightening) remain relatively unaffected at this stage.

Advanced Osteoarthritis of the Hip

There is no escape from the constant pain of a severely osteoarthritic hip. Sitting for any length of time is uncomfortable because it involves bending the hip. Bending is also involved in picking things up from the floor, so one is inclined to avoid that. Walking becomes extremely painful, as does going up and down stairs. Eventually the hip hurts even when lying down at the end of the day, when the joint is extended and not bearing weight.

Considering Surgery

Most patients manage to live with their osteoarthritic hip for a number of years. Then, gradually, as the pain increases, they may consider surgery. The actual decision may be triggered by the inability to tolerate anti-inflammatory drugs, a dramatic decrease in function, increased pain or pain severe enough to interfere with sleep.

The decision to have any surgery should never be taken lightly. A total hip replacement is major surgery, and though complications are rare, they do occur. Unfortunately, sometimes pain persists even after hip replacement. (See also Chapter 8, "Should You Have Surgery?")

The Operating Room

It is 8:30 A.M., and operating room 5 is full of activity. Six people clad in blue surgical garb, their faces covered with masks and their shoes with paper slippers, busy themselves around a short, seventy-two-year-old woman. Ines S. was born in Puerto Rico and came to New York with her husband and six of her seven children.

About ten years ago Ines developed joint problems. Her right knee gave her trouble. Arthroscopic surgery helped for a while, but after six years her surgeon decided to "fix her knee once and for all" with a total knee prosthesis, which to date has given her no problem.

Unfortunately, Ines's right hip then started to hurt. For a while routine medical care, including NSAIDs, exercise, and a cane worked, but eventually it became apparent that for Ines a total hip replacement (THR) was the most conservative course of action.

Because she had no other major medical problems, the admissions office scheduled Ines for same-day surgery. She had all her blood tests as an outpatient and talked to an anesthesiologist. Ines insisted on general anesthesia. In the weeks preceding her surgery, Ines was extremely nervous, and she arrived in the operating room full of apprehensions. She relaxed once she was premedicated with Versed (a Valium-like drug), and soon thereafter general anesthesia was induced. She also received antibiotics to forestall any possible infection.

Now Ines is fully wired to an electrocardiograph machine; the video monitor continuously displays her heartbeat and blood pressure. A catheter drains her urine into a flask, a respirator takes over her breathing, and a complicated vacuum system is ready to collect any drainage from the surgical wound.

Ines is draped in sheets except for her right leg, the target of the surgery. One of the surgeons scrubs the leg with a powerful antiseptic solution, encases it in a knee-high elastic stocking, and finally covers the entire surgical area with a plastic sheet lined with specially treated antiseptic gauze. The elastic stocking reduces the risk of developing blood clots during and after surgery. The chief operating room nurse arranges the instruments, sponges, and other tools required during the operation. At her request, the circulating nurse will fetch additional supplies from outside the operating room.

A light box near the operating table displays Ines's X rays. Her right hip exhibits signs of advanced osteoarthritis. The cartilage is almost completely gone, and the joint space is severely narrowed. Thirty years ago Ines would have had to live with this painful, nonfunctional hip. Now she has an option.

Ines S. lies on her side. A partition of blue sheets separates her head from her body. Her right leg is covered with an elastic stocking but can be moved freely. Her doctor, assisted by two other surgeons, makes a large cut in her side along a previously marked line. After the surgeons work their way through layers of adipose (fat) tissue, they finally reach the joint capsule.

Now the doctor can really examine Ines's hip joint. "The head of the femur is small," he notes, "and so is the acetabulum. I bet it'll take a small cup with a 22-mm inner diameter that will fit a 22-mm ball. Her osteoarthritis is far advanced—the joint space and much of the cartilage are gone. The head of the femur is full of pits and small craters." The surgeon asks for a paper measuring tape and measures the length of Ines's upper leg to make sure that the repaired hip will be the same length as it was before the operation.

Now it is time for the specialized cutting tool. The head of the femur is cut off, and the acetabulum is cleaned out. The surgeon reams it out with a rounded, circular drill head called an acetabular reamer and removes degenerated bone from the acetabulum. The drill heads gradually increase in size. Assistants use vacuum suction to keep the site of the operation as free of bone chips and other debris as possible. From time to time they wash the cavity out with saline solution. When the doctor is sure that the surface is clean, he measures it with spoon-like Charnley sizers. He tries several, but as he has predicted, Ines needs a small cup. This in turn dictates the use of a small (22 mm) femoral head.

The doctor decides to use a cemented prosthesis. The pros and cons of cemented or cementless implants seem to balance out (see later in this chapter). Surgeons anticipate very few surprises when using a cemented cup. Such certainty may not be true for the cementless procedures. The cemented cups are also simple to engineer, and less expensive. To affix the cemented cup, holes are drilled into the pelvic bone. These holes will accommodate the methylmethacrylate cement, which sets quickly in a warm environment and is ideal to anchor biocompatible materials like metal and plastic to bone.

When everything is ready, the surgeon asks the nurse to mix the methylmethacrylate cement. It hardens in fifteen minutes, so time is of the essence. The surgeons place the cup of the prosthesis into Ines's reamed-out acetabulum and hold it in place until the cement is set.

The surgeons now prepare Ines's femur. No osteoarthritic tissue has to be removed since the entire, partially degenerated femoral head has been cut off. Nevertheless, the hollow center of the femur, the femoral canal has to be carefully reamed out. As in the case of the acetabulum, some bone is removed to accommodate the methylmethacrylate cement that secures the stem of the new femoral head.

Everyone is busy. The surgeons call for retractors, saws, forceps, drills, sponges. The nurse, who by now looks like a conductor presiding over an orchestra, supplies these often before being asked.

Once the femoral canal is cleaned, the surgeon tries several classic Charnleys for size. (The hip prosthesis is named after the British surgeon who developed it.) When the doctor thinks he has selected the proper size, he bends and straightens Ines's new hip joint to see how it articulates with the acetabulum. He is very pleased with the way the head of the femur fits into the acetabular cup. The new joint, he feels, will be extremely stable.

The trial prosthesis is removed, and the femoral canal is carefully cleaned with an instrument that looks like a round dish brush. Extreme care is taken to insert the femoral stem just right. Before cementing the prosthesis in place, the surgeon again measures the length of the operated leg. It is the correct length.

Another batch of cement is mixed, and when it has the desired consistency, the surgeon inserts it into the prepared cavity of the femur. Then he inserts the stem of the prosthesis, taking care not to twist it as it goes in. When everything is in place, the surgeons inspect the pelvic cavity extremely carefully to make sure no debris remains. They now bend, flex, rotate, and twist the new hip. Everything works perfectly. The wound is sewn closed with self-dissolving thread. It will take from ten days to two weeks until the layers of flesh actually knit back together. A drain is inserted to remove fluid from the hip after the operation.

The surgery is over. The nurses pack up their equipment. Ines is clad in an ordinary hospital gown. A complicated pressure bandage encloses Ines's newly operated leg.

Ines is transferred to the recovery room, where her general anesthesia will wear off. This usually takes a couple of hours. Most patients are groggy or even nauseated. Backaches and headaches can occur after spinal anesthesia. When her vital signs are stable, and the staff is certain there will be no significant hemorrhage, Ines will be transferred to her room.

Recovery

During the first day or so, patients who undergo total hip replacement (THR) remain in bed. They often have considerable discomfort and may feel totally helpless. Some suffer from postoperative pain, and some experience backaches. Nevertheless, many people report that, for the first time in years, their arthritic hip is pain-free. In many hospitals a metal triangle hangs from a frame over the bed. By grabbing the triangle, patients can lift the upper portion of their body. This stretches the back muscles, exercises the arms and shoulders, and temporarily relieves stiffness and backache. Most doctors try to get their patients out of bed as early as possible. The stitches that close the wound will stay in place for another week or two.

To minimize the risk of blood-clot formation, both legs are now wrapped in elastic stockings. During the initial healing process the legs must be spread open. To this end patients keep a big pillow between their legs, even during sleep. This maneuver prevents dislocation ("popping out") of the hip from the socket.

♦ ♦ ♦ ♦ ♦ ♦ ♦

There is a lot of traffic in and out of Ines's hospital room. The surgeon comes once a day, as do the internist, several residents and interns, the head nurse, the day nurse, the night nurse, several orderlies, a dietitian, and the hospital chaplain. They check the IV drip, change the bed linen, provide a bed bath, deliver pills and food, and check Ines's temperature and blood pressure.

Sometimes, in spite of all this activity, nobody seems to be around when Ines needs a pillow adjusted under her hurting back or wants a glass of water or a book. For that reason she has hired a private duty nurse during these initial few days.

REHABILITATION (PHYSICAL THERAPY)

In the past, major surgery entitled patients to lie in their hospital beds just resting. This is no longer the case. Physical therapy starts within days after the operation.

Patients' reactions to physical therapy differ. Some patients are scared and need a lot of reassurance. Others, now free of the pain that kept them from doing things for months or years, are raring to go and have to be told to take it easy. Physical therapists spend a lot of time getting to know and educating their patients.

To begin with, many patients are afraid to stand up. After all, they know that their trusty old hip is gone. How can they be sure that their new one will hold their weight? Before they discover that it will, patients have to do some maneuvering.

Many people who have been flat on their back for twenty-four to forty-eight hours feel faint when they finally sit up. The feeling is partially caused by anemia resulting from blood loss and fortunately does not last. The blood-making tissues recover very rapidly after surgery, and the anemia passes of its own. It is, however, important to get up slowly to begin with.

After hip surgery this is easier said than done. It is important to keep the legs wide apart so as to prevent the hip from dislocating early on, before it has healed sufficiently. Getting out of bed without bending the hip and closing the legs is, however, quite difficult. To accomplish this feat, slide to the edge of the bed, keeping your legs apart. When you get to the edge of the bed, the physical therapist will help you swing your legs over the side. Sit up for a while to get your blood flowing, and only then stand up. To begin with you will use a walker.

Remember that the new hip is still very delicate and at first should not be bent more than 90° (a right angle). Some surgeons feel that the hip also should not bear much more than 10 percent of the total body weight at first.

These instructions puzzle many patients. How can they know what 10 percent of their weight is? Doing it is easier than it sounds. Your physical therapist may advise you to put half your weight on the walker, half on your good leg, and a little bit on the operated leg.

Once you are comfortable standing, try to take some first steps. Standard instructions provided by physical therapists are as follows:

- Stand firm on your good leg and divide your weight between the walker and the good leg, with only a little bit of weight on the operated leg.
- Transfer most of the weight onto the good leg and move the walker forward.
- Transfer most of the weight onto the walker and move the good leg forward. Divide the weight between the walker and the good leg.
- Move the operated leg to the level of the good leg.
- Repeat.

While you relearn to walk, the physical therapist will support your back.

The first day patients only take a few steps. Within days most patients walk well, and five days after the operation they usually proceed quite fast along the corridors of the hospital. Many now spend time out of bed, in the sun room, where the chairs are high and equipped with sturdy armrests so that patients can stand up easily.

Once you are out of bed, you can go to the bathroom. The toilet seat is elevated and has armrests. This prevents the hip from bending more than 90°.

Just when patients get used to their walkers, they must switch to crutches. Some surgeons prescribe elbow crutches. These do not fit under the arms like the regular crutches but snap around the upper arm. The crutches have a waist-level handle that is grabbed with the hands. Elbow crutches are lighter than under-arm crutches and relieve the armpits of some of the body weight. This in turn insures that there will be no stress on the nerves of the shoulder. Initially, elbow crutches are harder to use than under-arm crutches. Most patients, however, quickly become experts.

Once the operated leg is free of its cumbersome dressing, patients can move it more freely. Most patients worry about the loss of muscle tone. When stretched out flat, one cannot, for instance, lift a freshly operated hip even one inch. Such muscle weakness is quite natural, and in time, with gentle exercises prescribed by the physical therapist, muscle strength comes back.

Most surgeons postpone muscle strengthening exercises until after the six-week checkup. Then they provide their patients with appropriate exercises. Walking remains the best readily available, all-around exercise. It is important to be careful and cautious to begin with. One can hurt a new hip by using it too soon.

Once patients walk confidently with their crutches, they go to the physical therapy exercise room, where they learn how to navigate stairs. Again, it is important not to put the body's entire weight on the operated leg. This is how it is done:

Walking Upstairs

1. Put the good leg on next step.
2. Divide body weight between healthy leg and crutches.
3. Transfer operated leg to upper step.
4. Transfer weight to healthy leg.
5. Move crutches to the next step.

Walking Downstairs

1. Transfer operated leg to next step.
2. Put crutches on next step.
3. Transfer half body weight onto crutches.
4. Transfer healthy leg to next step.

Remember that the good leg leads up and the bad leg leads down. Before patients go home, the physical therapist may hand them a sheet of exercises.

Occupational Therapy

Before going home, patients visit the occupational therapy department. Here an occupational therapist teaches patients how to protect their newly operated hip during everyday activities. In order to avoid bending the hip, the occupational therapist supplies

- a plastic, raised toilet seat
- various gadgets to help with putting on shoes and stockings
- a long, scissorlike instrument with which to pick up objects off the floor (see Chapter 13 for details)

Going Home

After about eight to ten days, most patients are allowed to go home. They are told that they must live cautiously and carefully because it takes a while for a newly inserted hip to become stabilized.

After signing various papers, an orderly usually wheels patients to the door of the hospital. Then patients are on their own. They can go home by car or ambulette.

Because the hip should not bend more than at a right angle, it is difficult but manageable to enter an ordinary car. Since ordinary car seats are low, patients should sit in the front seat propped up high by a bunch of pillows.

During their first day or two at home, most patients are tired and many feel cross. Because of the crutches, it takes time to get used to the bathroom, the halls, the stairs. Many patients miss the comfortable chair they used in the hospital and may want to buy or rent one.

In order to prevent dislocation, the hip should not be bent excessively. Patients are cautioned

- not to overdo things
- not to bend their hip more than 90°, except to put on their shoes and stockings (this rotates the leg outward and is safe).
- not to sit on a low chair or, initially, on a regular toilet seat
- to take showers, not baths
- to sleep with a pillow between their legs.

Little by little patients get stronger. The new hip starts to feel wonderful and is totally or relatively pain-free. After about two weeks many have a hard time remembering to use their crutches.

Postsurgical Visit

About six weeks after surgery the patient returns to see the surgeon, who x-rays the new joint. The visit with the doctor is usually most pleasant. To check that the new hip works perfectly, the physician will watch the patient walk up and down the hall and then will cautiously bend, extend, and rotate the hip. Most often everything is fine.

Though two crutches are no longer necessary, patients are cautioned to let their hip heal for a few months. Some doctors recommend the use of one crutch for some time longer, then a cane for one month. Patients can now use an ordinary toilet seat and sit in a car without great worry. They are advised to avoid high-impact sports like jumping and running, and are reminded to take good care of their prosthesis—after all, it is man-made and can break down.

At the postsurgical visit surgeons supply their patients with a set of exercises that, when done properly, will improve muscle strength and flexibility. Walking remains the best all-around exercise. Swimming and water aerobics are also good, as are using an exercise bike or ski machine.

Minimizing stress also involves keeping one's body weight down as much as possible (for details, see Chapter 7, "Food and Osteoarthritis").

To reduce the possibility of the joint becoming infected, most surgeons provide their patients with a list of precautions. For example, antibiotics should be taken as directed before undergoing significant dental work (although recent studies question the need for prophylactic antibiotics before dental work) or any other invasive procedure (certain diagnostic tests, minor surgery). Any bacterial infection, even a bad sore throat, needs immediate attention.

New Developments

John Charnley's gift to the millions crippled by hip disease is so magnificent that any improvement pales in comparison. Nevertheless, the Charnley-type hip prosthesis has undergone some slight modifications.

Femoral Component

In the classic Charnley prosthesis, the femoral stem and the head of the femur were of one piece. In some hip prostheses the head can be a separate component from the stem. This permits a somewhat greater choice of sizes and allows for a more highly individualized fit. Older prostheses, however, have withstood the test of time and have certain advantages and, as we have seen in the case of Ines S., are still commonly used.

Cup

The acetabulum portion consists of a rather thick cup made of high-density polyethylene (plastic), which is cemented into place with methylmethacrylate cement. Other popular designs include cups that are part metal and part plastic and can be "jammed" into the bone and hold without cement. They are more expensive but can be inserted more quickly. In the long run, it is still not clear whether one approach is superior to another, and the debate continues.

Cementless Hips

Failures caused by the loosening of the stem portion of total hip prostheses increase with the number of years elapsed after the initial surgery. Since these complications were attributed to the methylmethacrylate cement, surgeons developed prostheses that do not require cementing. This alternative may be desirable for younger patients with a long life expectancy and, presumably, a very active lifestyle.

To enhance anchoring to the patient's bone, the metal components of the prosthesis have a porous (granular) surface. This meshwork provides a lattice designed to promote bone in-growth. Eventually this new bone fastens the prosthesis to the shaft of the femur and/or the acetabulum. To optimize this process, some implants are sprayed with hydroxyapatite, a bonelike substance. The surgeons may also fix the prosthesis into place by press-fitting it (jamming the prosthesis into its place in the bone).

One disadvantage of a cementless hip is a longer rehabilitation period. For bone-anchoring to occur, the joint must bear little weight

FIGURE 9-2: *Total Hip Prosthesis*

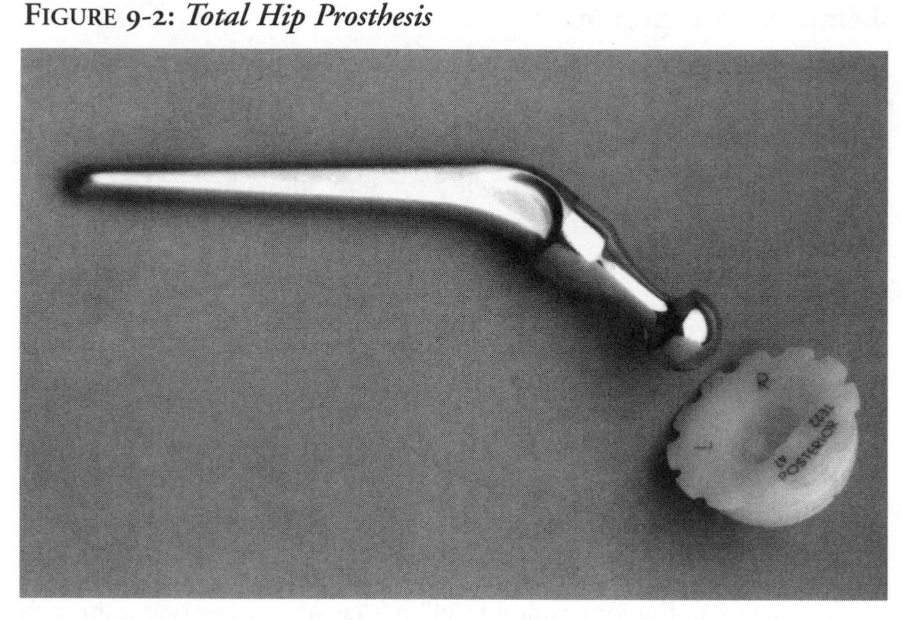

The total hip prosthesis is the oldest, most commonly used joint replacement. It essentially looks the same as the prosthesis developed by Sir John Charnley during the 1960s.

for six weeks or longer. This is another reason for younger patients to consider this option, since they have little trouble maneuvering with crutches. Older people may have a particularly hard time walking without putting much weight on the operated leg for that long.

Results with cementless hips have been mixed. Bony in-growth only occurs when the prosthesis fits very tightly into the femoral cavity. Human beings come in many shapes and sizes, and no two femurs are exactly the same. It is difficult to achieve a perfect fit with standard off-the-shelf prostheses. About 10 to 20 percent of patients with cementless hips report some pain in the front of the thigh. The cause of this pain is not always known, but it can be so severe that it requires reoperation. Another type of hip prosthesis is a cemented-cementless hybrid, in which the stem is cemented into the femoral canal while the cup is inserted into the acetabulum without cement.

A definite recommendation on whether to opt for a cemented or a cementless hip is not possible, especially since each patient's needs are different. As a patient you should take part in deciding what prosthesis to use. For example, do you want to stick with the old tried-and-true prostheses, or do you want to gamble on the latest developments? Your age may also be a factor. Discuss all the options with your surgeon; in the end he or she may have to make the final decision anyway.

COMPLICATIONS

Since the mid-1970s, total hip replacements (THR) have become common in the United States. It is thus not surprising that the number of second surgeries, or revisions, is increasing. According to National Center for Health Statistics, 25,000 hip revisions were performed in 1991.

Common complications encountered after total hip replacement are loosening, infection, dislocation, and wear.

Loosening

Aseptic (noninfected) loosening of a total hip prosthesis after it has worked well for a number of years can, unfortunately, occur. The initial sign of loosening is pain. A "radiolucent" or black line around the cement and bone may appear on a routine X ray.

There are many reasons for a prosthesis to loosen. The cement originally used to affix the prosthesis may weaken. It may also debond because of aging, osteoporosis, or widening of the central canal of the femur. The polyethylene cup inserted into the pelvic bone may wear down and shed debris. This debris in turn activates the immune system, which, in an attempt to remove the particles, will resorb bone, thereby accelerating the loosening process. Mechanical stress, especially in younger, more active, or heavier individuals, may contribute to the failure.

Infection

Among the most serious complications of THR are infections. Treatment often involves several surgical interventions, the outcome of which are sometimes disappointing to both the patient and the surgeon.

Infections that occur within six month of the initial operation may be caused by infectious organisms that, despite the many precautions, have seeded into the hip during surgery. Infection that occurs at a later date may have originated elsewhere in the body.

Infections can be chronic or acute. Chronic infections may go unnoticed for several years and come to light only when the prosthesis loosens. Acute infections, however, are never overlooked. They are extremely painful and often accompanied by fever, abnormal blood test results, pus, and other manifestations of virulent disease.

The first order of business is to identify the infectious agent. This is done by aspirating fluid from the hip joint with a fine needle and culturing this sample in the laboratory. Treatment is dictated by the nature of the infectious agents and the duration of the infection. In general, the joint is opened, cleaned thoroughly and drained. Unless the infection is very recent the implant must be removed. If cement is present, the surgeon will remove as much of it as possible. Antibiotics are administered intravenously for six or more weeks, because orally administered agents may not be strong enough initially. Some organisms are so virulent that treatment may last up to 12 months. Occasionally the infection may spread to bone adjoining the prosthesis (osteomyelitis).

Dislocation of the Hip

In about one percent of patients with THR, the head of the femur slips out of its plastic cup. Hip dislocations are extremely painful and can be recurrent. The danger is greatest during the weeks following the original surgery and then after about eight years, when the implanted components have worn down a bit. Most often dislocated hips can be reset without open surgery. The procedure involves realigning the two components of the prosthesis and immobilizing the joint for six weeks with a cast or a brace.

Conversions and Revisions

Patients with prior hip surgery may hear their doctor talk of "conversion" and "revision." The first of these refers to previously operated hips which now require *conversion* to a total hip prosthesis; the second is a *revision* (replacement) of a failed total hip replacement. In general, conversions, which often involve patients with a previous, healed, hip fracture, are less complicated than revisions. There can, however, be major exceptions to this rule.

Both conversions and revisions are much more complex and difficult than a first total hip replacement. It is essential that the operation be performed by a highly experienced surgeon, backed by an institution whose staff can provide individualized care including rehabilitation and treatment of deep-seated infections. Any intervention must be preceded by a careful presurgical evaluation. Enough blood for extensive transfusions and bone for grafting must be readily available.

The following factors must be considered prior to revision:

- Presence of a low-grade infection that requires detection and treatment before the surgery (see below).
- Extent of bone loss and need to augment the joint cavity with bone grafts. This does not require a separate surgical intervention. If the bone deficit is small, new bone can be harvested from the patient's own body. Larger grafts are obtained from regional bone banks.

Revision Surgery

As noted, unless identified very early, infection necessitates the careful removal of the prosthesis and of the cement anchoring it. Sometimes the old prosthesis is removed and replaced with a new one in a single operation. The new prosthesis is anchored with antibiotic-impregnated cement. The reported success rate of such interventions is 80 percent. Sometimes the infected prosthesis is removed, and reimplantation is delayed until the infection has been completely eradicated.

The surgery performed during reimplantation is similar to that previously described, except that it takes much longer—usually five to seven hours instead of two or three. This is taxing to both the patient and the surgeon. Moreover, there are special risks, as removal of the implant and of the cement can fracture the femoral canal. Newer techniques for cement removal utilize lasers (which vaporize the cement) or ultrasound. The ultrasound can be used to drive small cutting instruments or can be directly applied to the cement. This softens the cement, which can then be sucked out. Though the technique significantly shortens the time required for cement removal, it increases further yet the amount of sophisticated equipment required in the operating room.

Even though the removal of the cement is tricky, it is usually even more difficult to remove a solidly ingrown cementless prosthesis. The femoral cavity—which again may be so large that it requires bone grafting—is then fitted with a new cemented or cementless prosthesis.

Revision surgery requires flexibility on the part of the surgeon who must be prepared to modify the planned operative procedure as necessary. The complications that may occur during revision surgery are the same as those occurring during primary THR, except that their incidence is higher.

Postoperative rehabilitation after revision is completely individualized. Surgeons usually recommend that the hip joint be relatively immobilized for an average of six weeks after the operation. The more complex the surgery, the greater the length of immobilization during recovery. After revision patients are sometimes fitted with a short, single-leg, spica cast. Like a pair of cutoff shorts, a spica cast covers the hip up to the waist and goes down the thigh. Such a cast reduces the risk of hip dislocation and promotes healing of both bone and soft tissue. A short brace is also an option and can be used at the discretion of the surgeon.

Fracture of the Prosthesis

The stem inserted into the femur rarely fractures, but the bone itself can break. One patient with a successful THR felt so great that he decided to learn to ride a motorcycle. The first time he tried, he fell and shattered his femur. His new hip held, but setting the fracture was a major undertaking. A rod could not be inserted because the hip prosthesis was already in part of the canal. After months of treatment the patient finally managed to walk again, but not as well as before he broke his leg.

Hip Fractures

Total hip replacement is a true blessing for patients suffering from osteoarthritis; it is equally important for a fraction of the many elderly persons who break their hip. There are 300,000 hip fractures annually in the U.S., and according to the Bureau of Health Statistics, one woman in five will break her hip before her death. Setting these fractures with screws, nails, a side-plate, or performing a hemiarthroplasty (replacing half the hip joint only) is often adequate. Patients with certain types of hip fractures (femoral neck fractures, others) may be at risk of developing avascular necrosis (degeneration caused by inadequate blood supply to a particular tissue) or arthritis. Both conditions may require conversion to a hip replacement.

◆ CHAPTER ◆

10

The Knee

The knee is not an ordinary joint. As common parlance indicates, fear makes us feel "weak in the knees," and vanquished enemies are said to be "brought to their knees." Mechanically and functionally the knee is very complex. It folds upon itself, rotates, and locks when fully extended. Many parts of the knee, such as the kneecap and certain ligaments, are so complicated that their function and mechanism of action have only recently been understood. And there is still much to be learned.

THE ANATOMY OF THE KNEE

Bony Structure

The knee is the meeting place of the two longest bones of the body, the *femur,* or thighbone, and the *tibia*, or shinbone. The tibia is paralleled by a thinner bone, the *fibula*, which is not part of the knee joint. A small, round bone, the *patella* (kneecap), fits neatly in a groove (the trochlea) at the end of the femur and is the third bony component of the knee joint.

At its lower extremity the femur divides into two rounded knuckles called the *femoral condyles:* the medial condyle (medial means toward the center of the body) and the lateral condyle (lateral means toward the outside of the body). Both condyles move in unison with the top of the shinbone, the *tibial plateau.* The femoral condyles also move in unison with the kneecap, which acts as a lever, increasing the efficiency of the thigh muscles.

A look at the knee (Figure 10-1) shows that these three bones do not fit together as well as those of the hip. In fact, the ends of the bones seem to be mismatched: the femoral condyles are convex, but the tibial plateaus are not concave—they are flat, and sometimes even convex! A rubbery shock absorber called the *meniscus* fits snugly between the two bones and helps compensate for the mismatch.

There is only a thin layer of skin and fat over the knee joint. It is easy to see that the knee is a fragile joint. In addition to being vulnerable to twisting injuries, the knee is very susceptible to injuries from direct blows such as falls. Some physicians even refer to the knee as the "nightmare joint of the body."

Soft Tissues

Despite the poor anatomical fit of the bones, the knee is a most versatile and serviceable joint. The many ligaments, tendons, and muscles, along with the meniscus, insure mobility and stability.

Ligaments

These tissues connect bone to bone. Five ligaments play an important role in the knee. The *medial collateral ligament (MCL)* runs under the skin on the inside of the knee, the *lateral collateral ligament (LCL)* runs along the outside portion of the knee, and the two *cruciate ligaments—the anterior (ACL) and posterior (PCL)*—cross inside the knee. The MCL and ACL are commonly injured, and many an athlete will become familiar with them. Chronic injuries to the ACL can lead to abnormal motions between the femur and the tibia, which can then lead to arthritis. Finally, the large *patellar ligament* in the front of the knee attaches the patella to the tibia. Since the patellar ligament indirectly connects the quadriceps muscles to the tibia, it is referred to in common parlance as the *patellar tendon* (a tendon connects a muscle to bone). Osteoarthritis does not directly affect any of these ligaments. Arthritic deformities, however, can stretch out the collateral ligaments.

Cartilage

The top of the tibia and the bottom of the femur are cushioned by glossy, shiny, "glasslike" hyaline cartilage. In this as in other joints, cartilage serves as a shock absorber. It also provides a gliding surface

FIGURE 10-1: *The Knee: Bony Structure*

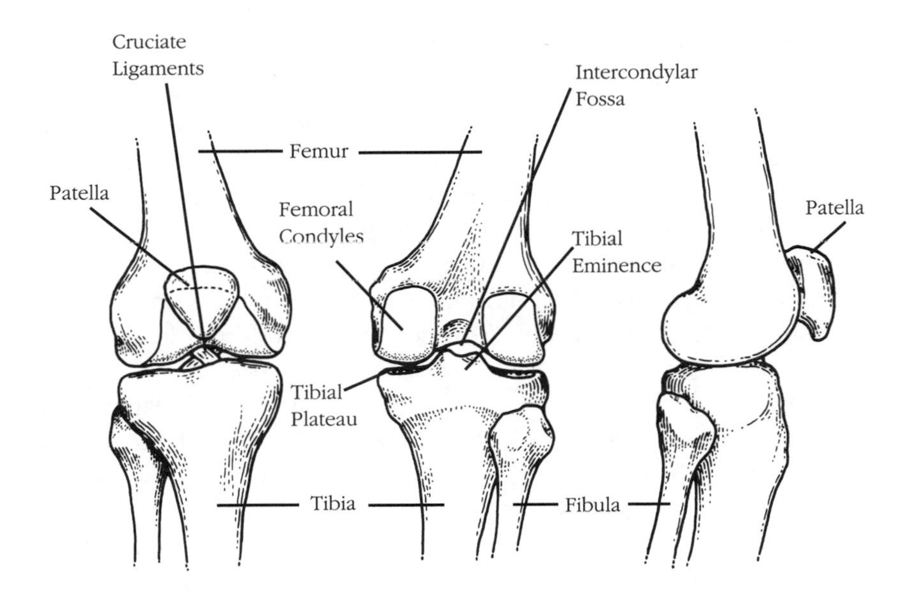

The knee joint connects the bottom end of the femur and the top of the tibia. At its lower extremity the femur divides into two rounded knuckles called the *femoral condyles:* the medial femoral condyle and the lateral femoral condyle. The rounded, depressed space between the two condyles of the femur is the intercondylar fossa.

The *tibia* (shinbone) ends in the *tibial plateau,* consisting of two shallow plates separated by two bony upward projections forming the *tibial eminence,* which moves with the *intercondylar fossa.*

A small, round bone, the *patella* (kneecap), fits neatly in a groove at the end of the femur and is the third bony component of the knee joint. The patella participates in knee motion, increasing the efficiency of the thigh muscles (quadriceps), which extend and straighten the knee. Stability in the knee is conferred by strong ligaments and muscles.

Two of the ligaments pass through the middle of the knee. Because they cross one another they are called the cruciates—from the Latin word *crux,* for "cross."

with minimal friction, which enables the joint to function smoothly and effortlessly. Osteoarthritis and rheumatoid arthritis attack this cartilage, causing it to pit, buckle, and gradually erode away.

Meniscus

The crescent-shaped menisci (the medial meniscus and lateral meniscus are commonly referred to as one unit), anchored to the top of the tibial plateau, shape themselves to the contour of the tibia and the femur. This conforming shape, along with the elastic nature of the tissue itself, partially compensates for the poor anatomic fit of the bones. The meniscus consists of rubbery fibro-cartilaginous tissue that is quite different from the smooth, hyaline cartilage covering the ends of the bones. In popular parlance the meniscus is often referred to as "knee cartilage," although this term generates some confusion.

Sport injuries and other trauma frequently damage or tear part of the meniscus. The meniscus has little blood supply and, like a broken fingernail, rarely heals. However, certain types of tears, especially in young people, can indeed repair themselves—either spontaneously, or with surgical help (see below). The injury to meniscal cartilage is very different from damage to the hyaline cartilage, a characteristic feature of osteoarthritis. Patients often are confused, however, because they are told they have a "cartilage problem," regardless of whether they suffer from arthritis or from a torn meniscus. If your doctor says you have a cartilage problem, ask for an explanation.

Joint Capsule

The knee joint itself is enclosed in a fibrous, baglike structure lined by a synovium. In a healthy knee the synovium secretes a small amount of lubricating fluid, the **synovial fluid**. After certain kinds of injuries the synovium may become irritated and secrete a large amount of fluid, much as the eye tears when it is hurt. An injured knee can feel swollen, hot, and heavy. It takes very little excess fluid for a knee to feel very swollen.

Bursae

Numerous small bursae (fluid-filled sacs) scattered about the knee tendons also provide cushioning and contribute to smooth movement. When a bursa is irritated, it fills with fluid and becomes painful. This is the familiar "bursitis." Bursitis also commonly occurs about the shoulder.

Muscles

These are the principle muscles of the knee:

- **Quadriceps:** the four muscles running down the front of the thigh into the knee joint. They straighten the knee and keep it from buckling when bending down.
- **Hamstrings:** the three muscles running down the back of the thigh—two on the medial (inner) side and one on the lateral (outer) side. The latter has two "heads" and is therefore called the biceps, as in the arm.
- **Gastrocnemius:** the muscle running along the back of the calf.

Bending of the knee is done by the hamstring and gastrocnemius; straightening by the quadriceps. When a physician taps the portion of the quadriceps between the kneecap and the shinbone (i.e., the patellar tendon), the knee quickly straightens. This is the familiar knee jerk physicians use to test the nervous system.

Rehabilitation after virtually any type of knee injury or surgery will include exercises to strengthen the quadriceps. Indeed, the dominant quadriceps may weaken and atrophy very quickly after injury or surgery.

The Three Compartments of the Knee

The knee is like an apartment with three connecting rooms:

- the *medial (inner) compartment,* which is towards the body's midline, or on the inside of your leg
- the *lateral (outer) compartment,* which is on the outside of your leg
- the *patello-femoral compartment,* which is the portion of the knee between the patella (kneecap) and the underlying femur.

Mobility and Stability

The knee is a highly mobile joint. It can bend 140°, closing upon itself like a jackknife. When the knee extends, it "locks" to become rigid, like a stick. The knee is not a simple hinge joint, however. The two condylar surfaces rotate with respect to the shinbone (tibia). When the knee is bent, the shin can turn right and left.

The knee is much less stable than the hip, which is a ball in a deep socket. The kneecap is particularly unstable. In some cases, it can be likened to a bar of soap gliding over another bar of soap.

Whatever stability the knee has derives largely from the ligaments and muscles that surround it. Thus, an injury affecting any of the ligaments or muscles weakens the complex joint and increases its instability.

Like the hip, the knee bears the entire weight of the body, and this stress increases severalfold during everyday activity. It is estimated that running, climbing stairs, and even getting up from a sitting position increases stress on the knee joint to several times one's body weight.

In a perfectly aligned knee, the weight-bearing force runs from the center of the hip through the center of the knee into the center of the ankle. Both the articular cartilage and the meniscus absorb a large portion of the load, and in a well-aligned knee, this load is well tolerated by the tissues. When a person is bowlegged or knock-kneed, the inner and outer compartments, respectively, take on a disproportionate amount of load and can wear out.

How Osteoarthritis Affects the Knee

One January morning, Philip B. got out of bed as usual and realized that both his knees were sore.

"It was a strange kind of pain," he remembers. "I thought that it might be some sort of rheumatism, and I paid little attention."

The pain, however, increased. Philip remembers that it became very intense whenever he started walking but subsided after fifteen to twenty minutes of activity. Curiously, if he sat down and rested for a while, the pain returned as soon as he resumed walking.

Philip tried several home remedies. Some helped a bit, but not much. Seven weeks later, in mid-October, Philip B. decided to consult an orthopedic surgeon. The diagnosis was clear-cut. Philip suffered from osteoarthritis of the knee.

It is surprising how often knees that have provided pain-free service for most of a lifetime seem to give out almost overnight. But osteoarthritis doesn't develop that quickly. Often a person's cartilage wears down in microscopic amounts until its thickness reaches a certain threshold. Then a joint, in this case a knee, suddenly stops functioning properly. Just a few weeks before knee pain crippled him, Philip had taken a long hike in the mountains and spent hours walking around Florence.

The initiating cause of osteoarthritis of the knee (and of other joints) is often unknown. Suspected triggers are malalignment (i.e., being bowlegged or knock-kneed), long-forgotten traumas and injuries, torn menisci, damaged ligaments causing instability, or old fractures. Improperly cared for injuries can eventually turn into chronic knee problems. Physicians now believe that inadequate treatment of an acute problem can be a common cause of osteoarthritis.

A certain degree of malalignment is present in most patients suffering from osteoarthritis of the knee. Like unbalanced automobile tires, improper alignment causes irregular wear of the cartilage. This results in a vicious cycle: the preexisting malalignment causes the osteoarthritis, which then leads to further malalignment, which in turn aggravates the arthritis.

Philip B.'s osteoarthritis most likely resulted from his being bowlegged. For fifty years the medial compartment of his knees bore some excess weight, causing the cartilage covering that part of the knee joint to wear out.

Thirty days after his initial consultation with the orthopedist, Philip B. checked into the hospital. The next morning, half of his right knee joint was replaced. Four months later, the surgeon replaced half of the left knee joint. Today, Philip is happy and looking forward to more hikes in the mountains.

◆ ◆ ◆ ◆ ◆ ◆ ◆

Dorothy O.'s decision to have knee surgery was almost as rapid. Her thickened and bent fingers made it obvious to almost everyone that she had osteoarthritis in other parts of her body. But though her knees had given her some trouble off and on through the years, they were still quite functional.

Dorothy had come to New York City from Allentown, Pennsylvania, during the 1950s. Big-city life attracted her, and she loved to dress up. Spike heels were a favorite accessory. She doesn't remember any notable injury but says she fell often. Periodically Dorothy's knees "acted up." When that happened, her internist gave her a shot of Novocain and/or cortisone. All that was many years ago.

Recently Dorothy fell while shopping. She seemed hurt but refused to go to the hospital. Instead she went home, applied hot pads, and used various other home remedies: pain relievers, vitamins, and food supplements. But her left knee never quite recovered. As is often the case, the fall did not cause the osteoarthritis, but it did precipitate the onset of symptoms. One day as she got out of bed, she found she could not bend her knee. Soon after, walking became almost impossible.

Dorothy consulted her family physician, who, after a thorough examination, sent her to an orthopedist. A thorough diagnostic evaluation showed that osteoarthritis affected all three compartments of her knee. Dorothy needed a total knee replacement.

Mild Osteoarthritis

Because of its inherent instability, the knee is the first joint affected in many patients suffering from osteoarthritis. Initial symptoms often include pain and stiffness upon walking and after a period of immobility, such as first thing in the morning or after working at a desk or watching TV for a long time. Initially the pain disappears when the knee is rested. The joint may also feel unstable. It may buckle suddenly, crack when it's bent, or give a snapping sensation. These symptoms are rather nonspecific and can be a sign of many other disorders. Diagnosis and treatment must be based on a more thorough evaluation.

Osteoarthritis often follows an erratic course. Many patients with osteoarthritis of the knee lead comfortable lives—especially if their pain is relieved by medication and they exercise regularly, rest when necessary, and avoid undue strain. In others, once osteoarthritis passes a "threshold," it progresses relentlessly. Then the pain rapidly becomes unbearable.

Many traumatic injuries result in immediate or long-term damage to the knee, which necessitates some of the surgical interventions described in this chapter.

The body's instinctive response to pain is to favor the unaffected part. The disuse of the affected part weakens the muscles and ligaments that contribute so much to the stability of all joints. The muscles surrounding the knee atrophy very quickly, and the "sick" knee can appear thinner than the healthy one.

Moderate Osteoarthritis

Progressively, osteoarthritis destroys the delicate architecture and function of the knee joint. The cartilage covering the ends of the tibia and femur wears away. The joint space narrows.

Severe Osteoarthritis

When the entire hyaline cartilage is gone and the joint space has vanished, bone rubs on bone, and any movement is excruciatingly painful. Large bone spurs, or *osteophytes,* may grow along the periphery of the joint. These spurs can be seen as the body's attempt to increase the area available for load bearing. They may also be the body's attempt to stiffen up the joint since less movement often means less pain. Depending on their location, these spurs can actually increase the pain.

Osteoarthritic damage is often limited to the destruction of the hyaline cartilage and the formation of bony overgrowths. There can also be a marked shortening of the tendons and ligaments, which makes it impossible for the patient to completely straighten the knee (*flexion contracture*).

Diagnosis

Treatment, including any surgical intervention, should always be preceded by a thorough diagnostic evaluation. This comprises a medical history of the complaint, a thorough physical examination, a laboratory workup, X rays or other imaging techniques (such as MRI), and a functional evaluation.

X Rays

A standard X ray outlines the damage wrought by osteoarthritis, including alterations of the joint space and the presence of bone spurs. As part of the workup, several X ray pictures are taken, showing the knee in various positions—extended, flexed, and especially weight bearing (standing). However, X rays may not pick up early arthritic changes, even if the pain is severe.

Functional Evaluation

When arthritis attacks the knee, there may be little correlation between X-ray findings and the actual pain and dysfunction. Treatment decisions are thus largely based on how much the pain interferes with lifestyle—how much the knee hurts at rest, when walking, climbing or descending stairs, or getting out of chairs.

During the functional evaluation the physician will want to know exactly how and when the knee hurts, whether an injury has occurred, and whether medication has been tried. Commonly asked questions include the following:

- Does your knee hurt (more or less) when getting up from a chair? (an activity that stresses the kneecaps), while you rest? (pain during rest indicates a more severe dysfunction), at night? when walking on stairs?
- Exactly what part of your knee hurts?
- Does the knee lock? (This can indicate loose pieces floating about the knee.)
- Does your knee feel swollen? (It will commonly feel so, even if swelling is not visible.)
- Have you ever injured your knee?
- Have you ever had injections for knee pain?
- Do any other joints hurt? (This might indicate rheumatoid arthritis or another systemic connective tissue disease.)

The physician will ask you to stand straight, to see whether you are knock-kneed or bowlegged, and walk, to see whether you limp or bend your knee abnormally.

Medical Treatment

The medical management of osteoarthritis of the knee differs little from that of other joints. First, you will minimize pain with anti-inflammatory or analgesic drugs (see Chapter 4). You will then be advised to follow these steps:

- Rest the knee as much as possible during acute flare-ups.
- Use ice when the knee is swollen or painful. (Some people prefer heat. Physical therapists usually advise patients to alternate

between heat and cold, and generally to do what feels best.)

- Exercise the knee appropriately and regularly (see pages 163–64 for specific knee exercises).
- Decrease physical stress on the knee by losing weight—or at least not gaining any (see Chapter 7)—and wearing well-cushioned shoes (see Chapter 13). Using a cane, walker, or golf umbrella can be helpful (for knee problems, the support can be held in either hand).

SURGICAL TREATMENT

Though doctors often try to delay total joint replacement operations as long as possible, Philip and Dorothy were advised to have knee surgery almost immediately, as their doctor felt that their osteoarthritis was far advanced and would not respond to nonoperative approaches. Though they had been unaware of it, the disease had progressed steadily until it suddenly interfered with their lifestyle. Philip could no longer take his usual long walks; Dorothy, who lives alone, had trouble taking care of her household.

Today knee surgery is so successful that surgeons use it much more readily than they did in the past. Still, any type of surgery represents a certain risk, and no patient should take the decision to have joint surgery lightly.

Two new developments, both perfected during the last two decades, have been good for patients with knee problems. The first is an instrument—the *arthroscope*—which permits surgeons to look inside the knee joint and to make small repairs. The second is *partial or total replacement of the knee surfaces.* Both techniques now complement older surgical procedures.

Arthroscopy

Arthroscopy, which uses a microscopic instrument, will be discussed later in this chapter.

Osteotomy

Osteotomy comes from the Greek and literally means "bone cutting." In the case of the knee, surgeons use the procedure to straighten out slightly abnormal bone structures such as valgus deformities, which may result in a person being knock-kneed, or varus deformities, which may result in bowleggedness. During the osteotomy the surgeon corrects the deformity by removing or adding triangular wedges of bone. An osteotomy is often used when arthritis is mostly limited to one compartment. For example, it may be highly suitable for bow-legged persons who have a tendency to wear out the medial compartment of the knee. An osteotomy will render them slightly knock-kneed, thereby possibly shifting the weight to the opposite compartment of the knee.

Osteotomies are useful when there is relatively mild disease, when the patient is too young for joint replacement, or if the repaired knee is expected to undergo major stress such as heavy physical labor or sports. There is still great controversy as to which patients are best suited for this procedure.

Fusion (Arthrodesis)

Arthrodesis means "fusion of a joint." In the case of the knee, it means fusing the ends of the femur and the tibia so they become one bone. Arthrodesis was once an accepted procedure to treat knee arthritis since it relieved pain. But a permanently rigid leg makes it difficult to sit in a car, a theater, an airplane or train seat, or any other narrow space. It also interferes with walking. Therefore, arthrodesis is seldom used today except in the case of certain infections or severe ligament loss when it is unsafe to implant a prosthesis.

Total Knee Replacement (TKR)

During a total knee replacement the surface layer of both sides of the knee joint are removed and replaced with man-made materials. Figure 10-2 shows a commonly used prosthesis. Because the knee is such a complex joint, it was difficult to develop a well-functioning prosthesis. Today most difficulties have been resolved. The procedure is quite safe and so successful that in the United States the annual number of total knee replacements exceeds the number of total hip replacements. To learn more about the procedure, let's follow Dorothy O. into the operating room.

The Operation

The day of her surgery Dorothy arrives in the OR in a wheelchair and climbs onto the operating table. Almost immediately Dorothy receives an injection of Versed (a Valium-like drug), and falls asleep, unaware of the bustle around her.

Everyone is busy. The anesthesiologists insert a tube down Dorothy's windpipe to connect her to the ventilator, which delivers air for her breathing and the precisely measured and closely monitored anesthetic. The anesthesiologists also run several leads from Dorothy's body to a monitor that will show her respiration, blood pressure, and heart function. They insert an intravenous fluid line into her arm to allow them to give her fluid and medication when necessary. They also insert a Foley catheter into her bladder to monitor urine output. The nurses wheel in several carts of sterilized instruments. In addition to small surgical saws, drills, forceps, clamps, sponges, and retractors, there are what seem like a whole hardware store's worth of knee implants. These are sterile trial sizes so that the fit of the final implant can be tried at the appropriate point during the operation.

A big light box displays the X rays of Dorothy's knee. Her doctor examines them repeatedly, evaluating the extent of the disease and reviewing with his team the optimal cutting angles.

A surgeon scrubs Dorothy's entire leg for fifteen minutes with a yellowish iodine solution. A specially treated plastic sheet is pasted to the area to be operated on.

To minimize bleeding during the surgery, a tight rubber stocking is placed on Dorothy's calf to empty the leg of blood. Blood inflow is then temporarily shut off with a tourniquet (a flat piece of inflatable material) placed around her thigh. Depending on the patient, it is safe to leave the tourniquet in place for an hour or two, making the operation almost bloodless. Finally, the entire leg is enclosed in a sterile stocking.

Dorothy breathes regularly. After an hour or more of preparations, everything is ready for the actual operation.

Overall Design of Knee Prosthesis

Legend has it that Cosmos and Damian, the patron saints of medicine, miraculously replaced the gangrenous leg of a faithful churchgoer with that of a slave who had died in a nearby bed in the same hospital. Cosmos and Damian were martyred in Rome in A.D. 330. Although true joint replacement came into its own some sixteen hundred years later, an early attempt at knee replacement echoes the technique attributed to the patron saints. In 1909 a surgeon transplanted the amputated knee of one patient into another who had lost his knee to sarcoma, a form of cancer. This was not a success.

Total (Bicondylar) Knee Prosthesis

Replacement with metal prostheses started during the 1940s, and many different hinged knee prostheses appeared during the subsequent decades. Once implanted, these prostheses were stressed by the normal movement of the knee, and most started to loosen within two years.

The major problems faced by surgeons and bioengineers developing a man-made knee were

- how to mimic the complex mechanics and motion of the knee itself
- how to preserve, as much as possible, the intricate system of ligaments, tendons, and muscles that provide the healthy knee with mobility and stability

After much trial and error Frank Gunston came up with a nonconstrained (unconnected, freely moving) prosthesis that proved moderately successful in the short run. Gunston's knee consisted of four nonhinged, separate parts: two metal semicircular femoral runners cemented into the femur and two high-density polyethylene tracks cemented into the tibial plateau. The four parts move in unison. The major drawback of the operation was the difficulty of aligning the four separate components.

Additional modifications resulted in the overall knee prosthesis design (shown in Figure 10-2), which most knee surgeons use today. This type of implant features the following:

- a femoral component, consisting of a metal alloy unit in which the two "runners" are connected by a metal strut; the entire component slips over the resected (cut down) condyles of the femur as if it were a huge dental crown.
- a tibial component, consisting of a metal plateau or tray attached to a stem, which is cemented into a hole drilled into

FIGURE 10-2: *Overall Design of Currently Used Knee Prosthesis*

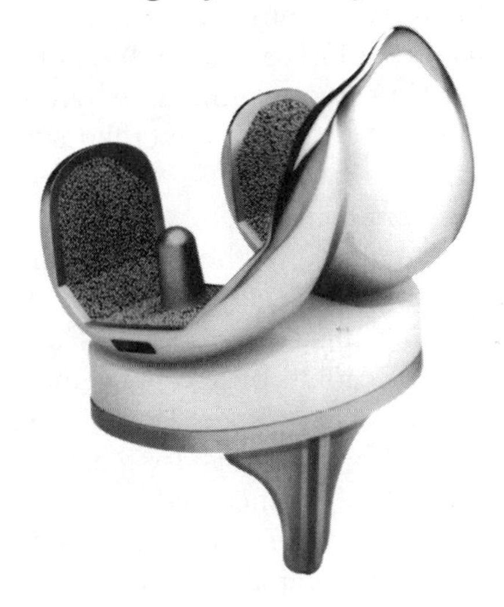

A total knee prosthesis. Note that the inside of the femoral component has a porous coating that permits the ingrowth of bone.

the tibia; this metal "tray" is surmounted by a high-density polyethylene plastic plateau, whose shallow sockets articulate smoothly with the metal runners of the femur; an additional polyethylene button covers the kneecap.

About 160,000 total knee replacements are performed in the United States annually. A remarkable number of knee implants are on the market, most of which have not been around in their present form for more than five years!

Among the various knee prostheses now in use, your surgeon will select the one that is most suitable for your condition, and one that he or she is familiar with.

Although a reconstructed knee bends only to 90°–110° instead of the "jackknife" 140°, the new knee prostheses allow for near-normal performance of daily activities such as walking, shopping, and even dancing.

Noncemented Knee Prosthesis

Since loosening of the cement is one of the major complications of total knee replacement, bioengineers are attempting to design prostheses that permit bone in-growth. Unlike cartilage, bone regenerates—otherwise broken limbs would never mend. When bone in-growth can occur, prostheses can hold without cement. Prostheses that permit the in-growth of bone have a rough, sandpaperlike surface at the metal-bone interface. It is hoped that their use will decrease the loosening problem, but this is far from guaranteed.

Recovery after a cementless prosthesis insertion takes longer than it would after surgeries using cement. Because the bone needs time to grow in, patients generally remain on crutches for three months or longer—as opposed to one month or less for cemented implants. The specific indications for cementless knee replacements remain controversial. There are pros and cons to this approach, and relatively little clinical data to evaluate. Most significantly, since it's such a new procedure, there are few long-term results available—the most important aspect in the evaluation of any implant.

Unicompartmental (Unicondylar) Knee Prosthesis

A good look at Philip's knees indicated that only the medial side of each joint was worn. He was an ideal candidate for unicondylar knee replacement.

Crude unicompartmental knee replacement operations were performed several decades ago but then fell into disfavor. Today a more sophisticated form of the unicompartmental operation is a good choice for patients with limited disease. A unicompartmental knee replacement—repairing either the medial or the lateral compartment—may be an excellent choice for young, active patients whose long life expectancy puts them at risk of outliving and outwearing their prostheses. Older patients, too, may benefit from this procedure if they are frail and would do better with less extensive surgery. These considerations, however, are still very controversial. Some surgeons, especially in the U.S., don't believe in the operation at all. Others reserve unicompartmental knees for older patients only. As in the case of the cementless prostheses, little long-term follow-up is yet available.

The less radical surgery required for the insertion of an unicompartmental knee prosthesis always spares both cruciate ligaments. Patients also have more flexion than with a total knee replacement and an almost normal perception of the position of their joints and limbs.

As with the total knee, many different prostheses are available for unicompartmental surgery.

A unicompartmental knee replacement is not simply half a total knee replacement. The two operations are actually quite different. Many surgeons have never performed a unicompartmental replacement and are unfamiliar with this operation. Take this into consideration when obtaining a second surgical opinion and choosing a surgeon. Unicompartmental knee replacements are usually less expensive to the hospital than total ones. This may be a significant factor in what is offered to the patient.

◆ ◆ ◆ ◆ ◆ ◆ ◆

Back to the Operating Room

After the over-an-hour-long preparation that followed Dorothy O.'s arrival in the operating room, her knee is now open and totally accessible. The surgeons can directly inspect the damage that the osteoarthritis has wrought. They remove all of the bone spurs and fatty tissue.

An electric saw cuts the femoral condyles and the tibial plateau. Holes for the stems of the prosthesis are drilled, planes are smoothed out. Because the knee capsule is tight, the surgeons must at times maneuver in a very narrow space.

The tibial side of the knee joint is readied first. After trying several tibial sizes, a size three is chosen for both the femur and the tibia.

Since this is a cemented knee, the nurse mixes the methylmethacrylate cement. Once mixed it must be used within minutes. The cement is carefully inserted into the hole that anchors the tibial stem and is spread over the tibial plateau.

The nurse mixes another batch of cement, and the surgeons cement the femoral condyles into place. The "button" for the patella is inserted. Then the surgeons bend the new knee back and forth. It seems to work fine. Everybody breathes a sigh of relief.

It is time to close up. Layer by layer the surgeon stitches the muscle tissue and the skin. A drain, which removes fluid from the wound, is inserted.

Including the time it took to set up, the operation has taken two-and-a-half-hours. The tourniquet is removed. Anesthetic administration is discontinued, and the anesthesia begins to wear off. The nurses slide

Dorothy carefully onto a special bed and wheel her to the recovery room, where she'll wake up and stay until the staff is sure that her temperature is normal and that her pulse and respiration will remain stable.

Time now to clean up the OR. The nurses examine all the instruments, scrubbing some and sending hundreds of items to be sterilized. Big, unopened instrument cases and the unused man-made parts are returned to storage. It is a full-time job to insure that every one of the many necessary instruments is readily available and in proper working condition.

Rehabilitation

When she finally gets to her room, Dorothy is ready to rest. She has arranged for a private registered nurse to take care of her that night. During the next day she plans to relax as much as she can, but her physical therapist has another plan. She comes to Dorothy's room and puts her "new" leg in a *continuous passive motion (CPM)* machine.

This machine gently bends and stretches the knee, allowing the joint to regain motion quickly. Its use is sometimes started in the recovery room or within one or two days after the operation. Initially the CPM bends the knee 20–30°. Gradually the range is increased, and after one week many patients achieve a flexion of 90°. The invention of this machine made a major contribution to the rehabilitation of knees after joint surgery, especially after total or partial knee replacement. The machines are so effective that some patients rent them for home use. Unfortunately, some insurance companies consider the CPMs a luxury, so you should make sure they will reimburse you.

Dorothy hated her CPM and dubbed it "the monster." Her doctor recommended using it twice a day, for a total of four hours. Other doctors recommend four to eight hours a day; others recommend still longer use.

Though she hated the CPM, Dorothy O. loved her physical therapist, who helped her sit up in bed, get out of bed, and walk with a walker, making sure she was safe and *felt* safe when learning to get around.

Most patients get out of bed two days after the surgery, but care must be taken to stand up *very slowly,* to avoid fainting. The physical therapist provides a walker and tells patients to put as much weight on their operated leg as they can stand. Soon thereafter, patients progress to elbow crutches, and finally to canes.

Going Home

Dorothy stayed in the hospital for two weeks and two days. This is a bit longer than usual. Six weeks after the operation she said that her knee was still swollen and achy. "Sometimes I have to use ice on it," she reported. She also complains that it takes her a long time to do anything. She still sleeps badly. An aide comes to look after her two hours a day and helps her walk to the dining room. She still uses her walker most of the time, but soon she can use her cane exclusively. She knows it takes three months to recover from this surgery. For several more months she may notice intermittent swelling of her leg. But day by day she does a little bit better.

Total Knee Replacement Exercises

Your surgeon will carefully prescribe the exercises he or she wants you to perform after total knee replacement, and your physical therapist will show you how to do them. In the beginning you will do these exercises a few times, two to three times a day. As you get stronger, each exercise should be repeated 10–15 times, two to three times a day.

Ankle Pumps

While lying on your back or sitting in a chair, pump your ankles up and down through their full range of motion. Repeat.

Gluteal Setting

While lying on your back, tighten your buttocks together, hold for a count of five, then relax. Repeat. This strengthens the muscles and helps straighten the knee.

Quadriceps Setting

While lying on your back, press the back of your operated knee down into the bed and tighten your thigh muscle. Hold for a count of five and then relax. Repeat.

Heel slides

While lying on your back, bend your hip and operated knee up while sliding your heel up the bed toward your buttocks. Repeat.

Terminal Knee Extension

While lying on your back with your operated knee bent and supported by a towel roll or pillow, lift up the foot to straighten the knee and then lower the straight leg slowly. Repeat.

Straight Leg Raises

While lying on your back with your nonoperated leg bent, raise the operated leg to the level of the bent leg (12–18 inches from bed) and then lower slowly.

Self-Assisted Knee Range of Motion

While sitting at the edge of the bed or in a chair, place a towel roll under your operated knee and bend it, while pushing it down with your nonoperated leg to assist. Repeat.

Knee Extension in Sitting

While sitting at the edge of the bed or in a chair, with both feet flat on the floor lift the operated leg (foot bent) until the leg is completely straight. Hold for a count of five, then slowly lower your foot down. Repeat.

COMPLICATIONS

Infections

As with hip replacements, infections are the most serious complication of knee prostheses. They occur in one out of two hundred cases even though great effort is made to maintain maximum sterility in the operating room.

Treatment of infections is similar to that discussed for hips. To begin with, a bit of fluid is removed, and the infectious organism cultured and identified. This permits an optimum choice of antibiotic therapy. After the knee cavity is cleaned in the operating room, intravenous antibiotics are started. Treatment lasts for three to six weeks. Intravenous antibiotics can be administered at home.

If such extensive therapy does not do the trick, the knee prosthesis may need to be removed. It can be replaced with a new knee, or the knee can be fused. It is usually a complex issue requiring a good discussion and rapport between patient and surgeon.

Stiffness

Some patients end up with a stiffer knee than expected. The first remedy is increased physical therapy. The doctor may prescribe a special splint in which a spring forces the knee to bend. Such splints can be worn for part of the day or night. Some patients require a "manipulation" in which, under anesthesia, the knee is gradually bent. As with any procedure, there are risks here, too (such as fracture). Surgeons disagree on the indications for such manipulations.

For additional details regarding complications, see also Chapter 9, "The Hip."

ARTHROSCOPY

Judy L. is very busy. Not only is she a physical therapist, but she is also the mother of three young children. Nevertheless it is rare that she does not go out for her twenty-minute run.

Now thirty-nine, Judy has been running since her mid-twenties. For a number of years she even ran marathons. Eventually the rigorous marathon training was too much, and Judy jogged simply to keep in shape and release everyday stresses.

Like most people, Judy has had her share of musculoskeletal problems. When she was nineteen years old, she had a triple fracture of the ankle. During her running career she had shin splints—a catch-all term referring to many different problems involving strained, overworked muscles of the lower legs.

Now, however, Judy seemed to have a more serious problem with her knee. First it felt funny when she jogged; then she noted a painful clicking when she exercised and/or ran.

Her doctor prescribed rest and an NSAID (see Chapter 4), and the knee got better. But Judy knew that there was something wrong. She consulted a specialist, who ordered magnetic resonance imaging (MRI).

This diagnostic technique can be a helpful procedure because, unlike a traditional X ray, which only shows bone, an MRI "photographs" soft tissue.

Judy's MRI suggested that she might have a tear in the meniscus. Arthroscopy was recommended.

The Instrument

An arthroscope is a fiber-optic instrument consisting of bundles of extremely thin, coated glass fibers. These fibers transmit light from one end to the other. Arthroscopes permit doctors to inspect joint surfaces directly, in living color and motion. This allows for a more accurate diagnosis, especially of disorders involving the soft tissues, and enables the physician to visualize small localized lesions.

In addition to arthroscopes for joint inspection, fiber-optic instruments include laparoscopes for exploring the abdominal cavity, and endoscopes and sigmoidoscopes for investigating the intestinal tract. When they were first developed during the 1950s, the primary use of fiber-optic instruments was diagnostic. Since then, however, the instruments have become equipped with tiny graspers, scalpels, shavers, burrs, and suction devices to carry out many surgical interventions that previously required more invasive surgery.

Arthroscopy is most often an outpatient procedure. The instrument is small—only 4 mm in diameter. Its insertion into the knee requires only a very small incision, which usually requires at most a single suture after the procedure is over.

In the case of the knee, the arthroscope is most often used to address small tears in the meniscus. The instrument is also used for joint debridement (removal of accumulated debris). These procedures usually require snipping off fronds of articular cartilage hanging from the bone like paint from a peeling ceiling, or removing other useless tissues, including loose bodies and osteophytes that interfere with the knee's proper function.

The Procedure

Even though arthroscopy is considered by some to be minor surgery, it carries some of the risks of more extensive procedures such as residual stiffness, infection, pain, or reaction to anesthesia.

FIGURE 10-3: *The Arthroscope*

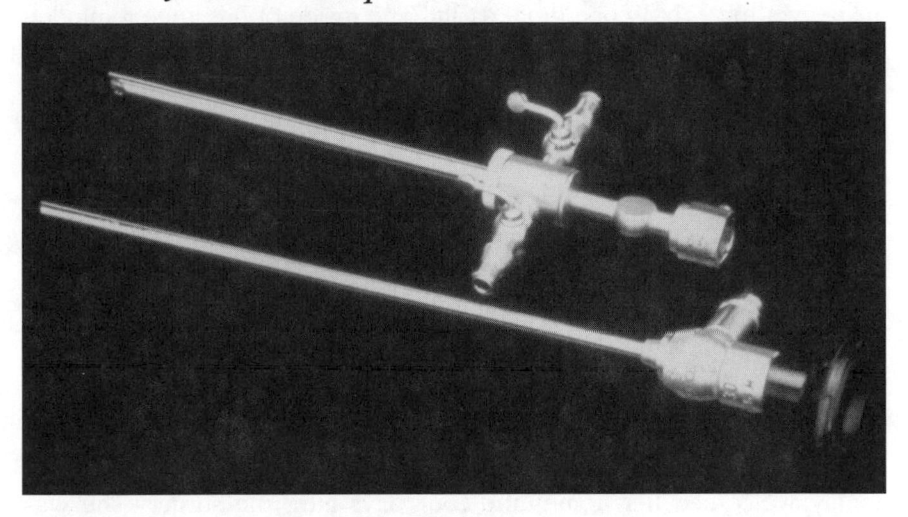

An arthroscope is a fiber-optic instrument developed to look into joints. Today its use in surgical procedures allows for minimal incisions.

A few days before the surgery Judy had her presurgical blood tests. The morning of the surgery Judy went to the hospital, was assigned a locker, undressed, and put on a surgical gown. A nurse carefully shaved her knee. Then Judy walked into the operating room, climbed on the operating table, and was given an epidural anesthetic. The anesthesiologist injected a local anesthetic into in the epidural space (a padded layer surrounding and protecting the spinal cord) in the lower back, which numbed the nerves from her waist to her toes. Judy also received some Versed. An intravenous line was inserted into her arm just in case there was an unlikely emergency, and general anesthesia was required. Electronic monitors continuously recorded Judy's blood pressure and heart rate. The anesthesiologist could also have opted for strictly local or for general anesthesia. Patient preference plays a role here. (See Chapter 8 for a discussion of anesthetics.)

After a few minutes Judy's entire leg started feeling numb, but she could still wiggle her toes and was worried she would feel the arthroscope entering her knee. The surgeon told Judy not to worry, and indeed she did not feel anything. Her leg was shielded, so she could not see it, but she could watch the entire procedure on the television screen.

To begin with, the surgeon injected some fluid so that he could maneuver the arthroscope more easily. The inside of her knee reminded Judy of outer space. The ends of the bones were very white and looked like planets. The muscles were red. The entire cavity was filled with fluffy stuff that looked like cotton. "That's degenerated cartilage," the surgeon told her.

The surgeon moved the pencil-like arthroscope around the inside of Judy's knee, cutting and vacuuming all at the same time. He noted that her anterior cruciate ligament looked good. He also saw that the meniscus indeed had a small tear. After thirty minutes the procedure was all over.

The entire lower portion of Judy's body now felt paralyzed. A nurse wheeled her into the recovery room where she dozed, on and off, for an hour and a half. When she woke, it was time to go home. Her knee hurt, but not too badly, and she used a cane to get into the taxi. Her family welcomed her home, and four days after the surgery she was ready to go back to work.

The Outcome

The tear in Judy's meniscus was smaller than expected, and for the time being the inside of Judy's knee is nice and clean. Unfortunately, the surgeon discovered that her knee articular cartilage was a bit damaged—a very early indication of OA of the knee. When someone has a small area of cartilage wear (early osteoarthritis), it is difficult to predict the progression of that lesion. It may progress and the area of wear may increase. This can lead to increased pain. On the other hand, the area of wear may remain unchanged over time. For the moment it is not possible to predict which lesions will deteriorate further and which will remain unchanged. Even though the damage might have been there for a while, the surgeon advised Judy to cut down on her jogging, and Judy is most unhappy. However, her knee has healed nicely, and for now she is as good as new.

◆ CHAPTER ◆

11

The Back and Neck

THE BACK AND ITS PROBLEMS

References to the back are common in everyday speech. The courageous have "backbone," the unpleasant are a "pain in the neck," and the cowardly are "spineless."

The spine is very central to the anatomy. It holds up the entire body, provides structure and support, and allows humans to walk erect. In addition, the spine or vertebral column houses the spinal cord, the body's principal communication channel.

Until approximately twenty years ago, diseases involving the human spine were among the most difficult problems in orthopedics. After the common cold, an ailing back is America's most frequent cause of absenteeism and disability. Both patients and surgeons were reluctant to resort to back surgery for a host of reasons.

The medical and surgical care of the back improved markedly during the 1980s. Diagnostically, physicians were able to pinpoint more accurately the possible cause of a back problem and to predict with some certainty whether surgery would resolve it.

Before these diagnostic developments, back surgery was often unpredictable. People with back pain might, for instance, be advised to have a disk removed. Often this procedure did not eradicate the pain. Instead of acknowledging that the disk was not the sole problem, health professionals implied that the pain was "all in the patient's head" or that they were malingering. The many failures branded back surgery with a very bad reputation.

Today new imaging techniques help clearly identify the source of the discomfort. These developments are particularly important for persons suffering from arthritis. For instance, orthopedists are now able to differentiate a slipped disk from arthritic changes in the surrounding bone.

The Anatomy of the Back

The Bony Structure

The spine is the longest bony structure of the body. It is intricately constructed to provide both stability and mobility. The spine consists of twenty-six separate vertebrae interconnected by muscles, discs, cartilage, and ligaments.

Each individual vertebra (Figure 11-1) has an intricate structure. Its main portion consists of a thick slab of bone, which bears the brunt of the body weight. To accommodate the blood vessels that supply the bone with nutrients, each vertebra is pierced by several passages, including the nutrient *foramen* (foramen means opening or passage). The cartilaginous end-plates of the vertebra (its upper and lower surfaces) facilitate the attachment of the intervertebral disks. The back portion of the vertebral body is curved and forms the front part of an arch, which extends toward the back of the vertebra, forming a well-protected central space. This canal, the *spinal canal*, accommodates the spinal cord and the nerves.

Processes (bony extensions) arise from the vertebral arch. These downward projecting bones are so arranged that the vertebrae overlap with one another like stacked flower pots. The fit is so tight that the spine is often called the spinal or vertebral *column*. A complex system of muscles and ligaments connects the bony processes (projections) of the spine to one another. When viewed from the side, the normal spine has three curvatures: the cervical curve (neck), the thoracic curve (chest), and the lumbar curve (low back).

FIGURE 11-1: *The Vertebrae*

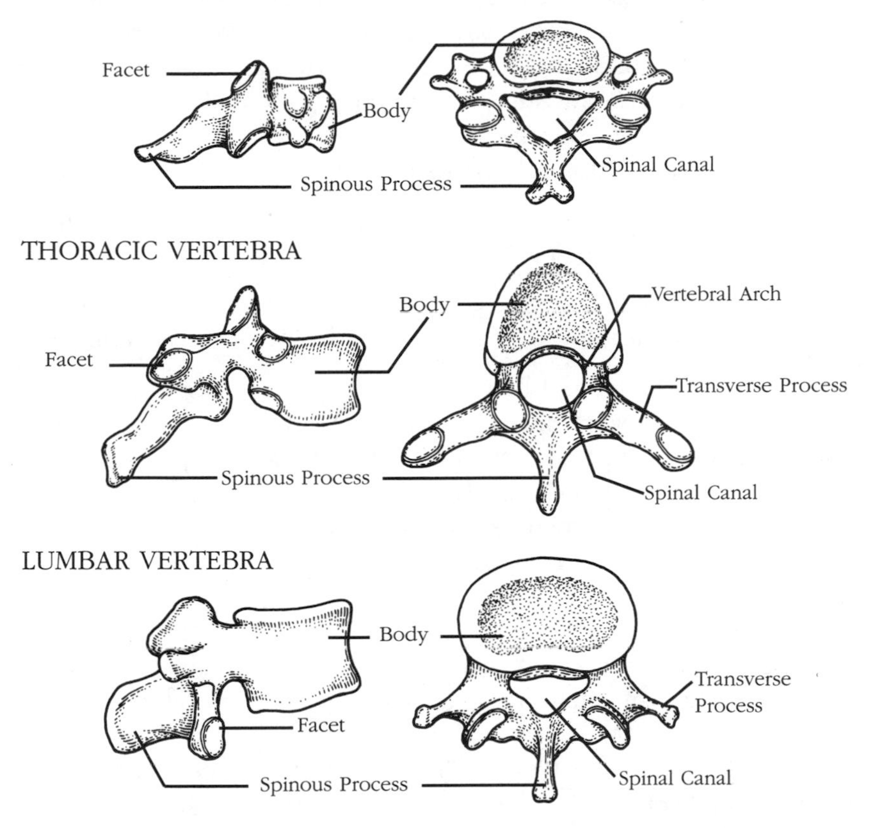

The spinal column consists of twenty-six individual vertebrae. The vertebrae are very complex, enabling the back to fulfill its three principal functions: protecting the spinal cord, providing rigidity, and allowing mobility. The body of each vertebra consists of a thick, bony slab pierced by a number of tunnels and grooves, permitting the passage of nerves and blood vessels.

Several bony processes (projections) extend from the back of the vertebra. One of the bony extensions, the spinous process, extends straight backwards, giving the spine its typically knoblike appearance. Two bony processes project downward, enabling the vertebrae to stack tightly, one on top of the other, like nesting flower pots. The surfaces of these articular processes—the facets—form true synovial joints between the vertebrae.

The vertebrae are separated by intervertebral discs. These shock absorbers consist of a fibrocartilagenous core filled with a pulplike, softer center. There are differences between cervical, thoracic, and lumbar vertebrae.

The Soft Tissues

The vertebrae themselves are attached to one another by the intervertebral disks. These function as spacers and shock absorbers. In a healthy spine the disks allow for smooth movement and maintain the proper distance between vertebrae, protecting the delicate nerves from pressure as they exit from the spinal canal.

Each intervertebral disk consists of

- a very tough outer shell, the *annulus fibrosus,* that firmly anchors to the vertebra
- a softer, semiliquid center called the *nucleus pulposus,* which allows the entire disk to behave like a hydraulic ball-bearing

In order to attract and bind water, the *nucleus pulposus* is rich in proteoglycans, whose chemical constitution allows them to bind a large amount of water. The water content of the *nucleus pulposus* increases the resilience of the entire disk. The elastic intervertebral disks ease the loads that weigh on the spine and distribute them in such a manner that the pressure exerted on any one portion of the vertebra is minimized.

As Figure 11-2 (the spine) shows, the intervertebral disks connect the vertebra on their anterior (front) side. On the posterior (back) side, the vertebrae are attached to one another through special joints, called *facets.*

The facet joints are typical diarthroidal joints (see Chapter 3) in which the ends of the bone are covered with smooth, slippery hyaline cartilage. The entire joint is enclosed by a joint capsule and lubricated by synovial fluid. As always, the healthy articular cartilage is highly polished, permitting pain-free movement.

The Vertebral Canal and the Spinal Cord

The vertebral canal protects the spinal cord—the lower portion of the central nervous system (CNS). The spinal cord contains both gray matter, a major constituent of the brain, and white matter. Gray matter consists mostly of interconnected nerve cells that carry out many of the functions of the brain. White matter refers to nerves enclosed in a myelin sheath. More specifically, the white matter of the spinal cord consists of many pairs of spinal nerves that emerge from both sides of the cord to innervate various portions of the body: the trunk, the arms, and legs. The spinal cord thus functions like the principal cable of a large telephone network.

The gray matter of the spinal cord extends from the brain to the beginning of the lumbar region (L1 or L2). The presence of gray matter in the upper regions of the spine makes back injuries and surgery at the level of the neck and upper spine inherently more risky than those affecting the lower back.

Soon after leaving the spinal cord, each spinal nerve root divides into sensory nerve fibers and motor nerve fibers. These sensory nerve fibers transmit sensory input from the skin and muscles *to* the brain, and motor fibers send messages *from* the brain to the muscles, glands, and other effector organs. Both sets of nerves continue to subdivide as they distance themselves from the spinal cord.

The spinal nerves leave the spinal cord through specific short tunnels or nerve canals on each side of a vertebra. These are the *right and left neural foramina.* As we shall see, these nerve canals play an important role in degenerative diseases.

Overall Structure of the Spine

The vertebrae are subdivided into four regions (see also Figure 11-2):

cervical (C) (seven vertebrae)

thoracic (T) (twelve vertebrae)

lumbar (L) (five vertebrae)

sacral (S) (five vertebrae)

The sacral vertebrae are usually fused together.

In each section, the vertebrae are numbered top to bottom beginning with one. When a physician refers to a problem as L3–L4, he or she is talking about the intervertebral disk in the lumbar spine between vertebrae 3 and 4.

FIGURE 11-2: *The Spine*

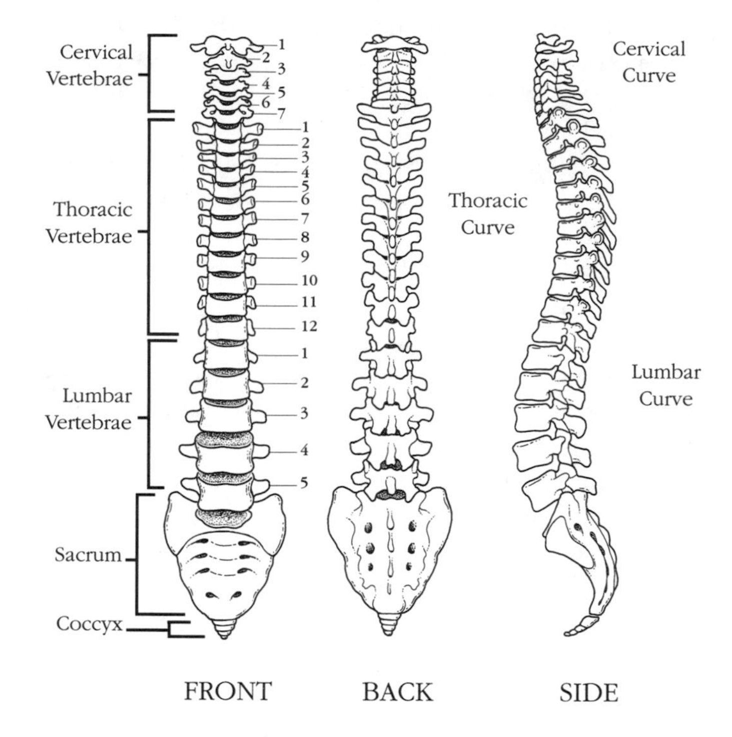

Here are three views of the spine. The intervertebral disks, which connect the vertebrae on the anterior (front) portion, are best seen in the front view here.

The long extensions of the transverse processes are best seen in the posterior (back) view.

The curvatures of the spine and the spinal processes are shown clearly in the side view.

Also note the numbering and the vestigial tail (coccyx).

The Cervical Spine

The uppermost portion of the spine is the cervical spine, or neck. It consists of seven small vertebrae. The topmost cervical vertebra (C1) is ring-shaped, devoid of bony processes, and very mobile, enabling people to nod and shake their heads. Since it carries the head, C1 is aptly called *atlas,* after the Greek hero who carried the world on his shoulders.

The Thoracic Spine

The thoracic spine occupies the chest region. It consists of twelve vertebrae, each of which is attached to two ribs. The ribs and the nature of the intervertebral joints make this region of the spine rather rigid. This is why it exhibits fewer osteoarthritic changes and fewer disk problems.

The Lumbar Spine

The five vertebrae of the lumbar spine are in what is commonly called the low back. They are bigger and heavier than those of the neck and thoracic spine. Because they are lower down, they carry a proportionately larger share of the body's weight. These vertebrae are highly stressed and more susceptible to degeneration.

The Sacrum

The sacrum is a triangular bone formed by the fusion of five sacral vertebrae. The sacrum, located between the two iliac (hip) bones, is part of the pelvic girdle.

The Coccyx

The coccyx, the vestige of a tail, is also triangular. It is the rather rudimentary end of the spine.

Motions of the Spine

The mobility of the spine arises from a complex interplay of the facet joints and the disks. As everyone with a sore back knows, the spine seems to participate in almost all physical activity: walking, standing, sitting, running, swimming, and so forth.

The special orientation of the facet joints, which varies with each region of the spine, governs overall mobility. The lumbar spine, for example, moves forward and back (flexing and extending) while allowing only a certain amount of twisting. The cervical spine, on the other hand, is much more mobile—flexing, extending, and rotating.

Degenerative Diseases of the Spine

Who Has Osteoarthritis of the Spine?

People attach great importance to their back. A diagnosis of spinal osteoarthritis generates greater fear than, for example, one of osteoarthritis of the hip. Actually, osteoarthritic changes of the neck and lumbar spine are quite common—one study indicates that it affects 60 percent of people over sixty. But these degenerative changes do not always result in clinical symptoms.

To a large extent spinal osteoarthritis is related to lifestyle. Extended sitting, for instance, promotes osteoarthritis of the lumbar spine. Cigarette smoking, alcohol consumption, and weight gain are also thought to promote spinal osteoarthritis. The harmful effects of cigarette smoking might be due to undesirable vascular changes in the blood vessels that supply the spine with blood. Cigarette smoking also slows the recovery from spinal surgery.

But in general the osteoarthritic processes affecting the back and neck are probably not all that different from those occurring elsewhere. The initiating cause is usually not specifically known.

Once the process starts, there is a disruption of the smooth movement of the joint, an unsuccessful attempt at repair, and finally overall interference with pain-free movement. Because the back is so complex, however, the consequences of osteoarthritic changes may be quite varied.

The osteoarthritic changes of the spine also may be a consequence of the normal, slight asymmetries of the human body. With aging, normal variations in leg length or a minor spinal curvature may cause stress that eventually causes degenerative changes.

In general, the various osteoarthritic processes that affect the spine cause one or more of the following problems:

Compression (squeezing, stenosis) of the nerve roots as they leave through the nerve canal.

Malalignment of the spine caused by the loss of its intricate architecture. Malalignment interferes with normal twisting and tilting movements and can also alter the existing curvature of the spine. This in turn can lead to additional degeneration and pain.

Instability of the spinal column. Wear, resulting in tissue loss, may increase the mobility between two or more vertebrae. The resulting instability causes stress, which in turn can trigger degenerative changes.

Common Osteoarthritic Changes of the Spine

Facet Joints

The facet joints that connect each spinal process with the one directly beneath it are typical joints consisting of cartilage, joint space, and joint capsule. As Figure 11-1 shows, these facet joints are in close proximity to the *neural foramina*, through which the nerves leave the spinal cord.

Wear and tear can result in cartilage degeneration, which in turn can result in osteoarthritis characterized by an uneven joint surfaces. Typically the underlying cartilage becomes denuded and pitted. This may trigger a repair process and the formation of osteophytes or bone spurs. As the disease progresses, the facet joints become larger than normal. These enlarged facet joints can reduce the size of the opening of the *foramina*. Such narrowing, called spinal stenosis, compresses the nerve root, causing pain and numbness or weakness. Depending on the precise site of the stenosis, the pain may be felt in the arms, legs, or elsewhere.

The Intervertebral Disks

With wear and tear, age, or trauma, the outer layer of the intervertebral disks may develop some cracks, and their perfectly sealed softer centers may dry out. As these alterations progress, the disks may collapse, increasing the pressure on the body of the vertebrae, which may respond with bony overgrowth and osteophyte formation.

Sometimes a fissure in the tough outer shell of the intervertebral disk may cause its soft center to bulge out, or herniate. This condition is referred to as a *slipped disk.* This term is a misnomer, since nothing actually slips. Calling the condition a herniated disk is much more accurate. In any case, once the jellylike inside of an intervertebral disk leaks out, it presses on the adjoining nerves, causing intense pain that could even result in nerve damage.

Osteoarthritis of the Neck

Symptoms of this common form of osteoarthritis are varied. People often first note a certain tightness when turning their head and looking back over their shoulder. In addition to stiffness, patients may also note headaches, shoulder pain, weakness of the arms, face pain, or staggering gait.

Secondary Osteoarthritis

Osteoarthritis often develops at the site of an old injury or preexisting deformity. A case in point is scoliosis. In scoliosis the spine is curved to one side or the other when viewed from the back. Scoliosis can be so severe that it requires surgery, or so mild that it goes unnoticed. Some scoliosis patients who have had successful back operations during their childhood or in their teens develop secondary osteoarthritis at the ends of their scoliosis fusion.

Synovial Cyst Formation

Cysts filled with synovial fluid occur occasionally in a variety of joints. When they occur in the spine, which is very rare, they may become quite bothersome.

DIAGNOSIS

Inaccurate diagnosis is one reason that back surgery used to be so problematic. Back pain is often so unspecific that a detailed diagnostic work-up is crucial. It is important to remember that pain originating elsewhere (kidneys, ovaries, hips, or shoulders) is often referred to the back. If all commonly used diagnostic techniques—physical examination, X rays, and imaging—concur, then your doctor can be reasonably certain that the nature of the problem has been identified.

On the other hand, if the results are ambiguous—for example if the patient complains about pain on the right side and the CT scan or X ray indicates a left-sided irregularity—the cause of the problem is less certain.

Types of Back Pain

Three types of back pain are most common:

Lumbago pain: A dull pain in the low back region, which increases from the buttocks to the back of the leg, often into the foot during standing and sitting.

Sciatica pain: A sharp, radiating pain shooting down the buttocks, thighs, or legs.

Neurogenic Claudication: This cramplike pain characteristically develops after minor exertion. For instance, leg cramps may develop after walking for a short distance, forcing the person to stop. The term *claudication* is classically used in conjunction with vascular insufficiency and usually indicates an insufficient blood supply to a working muscle. In the case of the back, claudication can be due to a narrowing of one of the many bony canals through which the blood vessels that supply the spinal nerves pass.

Medical History

Diagnosis always starts with a detailed medical history. In the case of the back, the emphasis will be on recent or former accidents (such as whiplash injuries or falls), occupation and hobbies, any unusual emotional stress, and the level of pain and its patterns.

Physical Examination

Even though the causes of back pain can be varied, a thorough physical examination may nevertheless indicate the pain's origin. To examine the back, most orthopedists adhere to a systematic approach:

- **Overall inspection of the neck and back:** This would include checking leg length (both should be about equal) and palpating the back while the patient is lying down or standing. A sharp pain in any portion of the back may help pinpoint specific problems. The exam may also reveal any preexisting, previously symptomless misalignment such as scoliosis.
- **Gait, posture:** Back pain, even when minor, usually affects the manner in which people walk and stand. The doctor will watch as you walk or stand.
- **Mobility:** This evaluation includes forward flexion (bending), lateral flexion (bending sideways), chest expansion, squatting, rotation, and hyperextension (bending backwards).
- **Muscle strength:** Muscle strength is as important as mobility. Physicians go to great lengths to evaluate the strength of the legs and feet. For example, straight leg raises are usually painful for patients suffering from sciatica. A major difference

in the circumference of the two thighs or the two calves (both should be roughly equal) indicates that one leg is weaker, possibly because of nerve damage or neglect.

- **Reflexes:** Testing includes the familiar knee jerk as well as the ankle jerk.
- **Sensation:** During this test the physician touches various areas such as the leg and foot with sharp and soft objects. Responses may implicate or exclude involvement of a particular area of the spine.

A detailed physical examination may enable the physician to diagnose a back problem and often provides sufficient information to initiate medical treatment. The following techniques are used when the diagnosis is unclear or if surgery is contemplated. They are expensive, however, and should be used only if strongly indicated.

Myelography

The diagnostic developments of the last 20 years have not only enabled orthopedists to make a better diagnosis, but have also abolished much of the discomfort associated with the in-depth evaluation of back disorders. Take for example a myelogram, which is a type of X ray of the spinal structures. This test involves injecting a dye into the spinal sac. The dye outlines the intervertebral disks, obstructions, nerve root injury and other soft tissue abnormalities not visible on a plain X ray film.

In years past, the dye was oil-based and irritating and could not be excreted by the body. The dye thus had to be removed by aspiration. The entire procedure required hospitalization and was accompanied by nerve root irritation, headaches, nausea, and vomiting.

Today the contrast medium is a water-soluble dye, which is eliminated by the kidneys. Unpleasant side effects occur much less frequently.

Computerized Tomography (CT Scan)

This procedure combines computer technology with X rays. By taking a series of X rays at different angles and feeding the results into a computer, the CT scanner provides the physician with cross-sectional and three-dimensional images. This technology, available since 1972, is especially valuable for soft tissues like the brain or for tumors that do not show up on ordinary X rays. Computerized tomography is also particularly helpful for structures like the spine, in which changes in the soft tissues (nerve roots, cartilage, and disks) may contribute heavily to the dysfunction. CT scans also provide an excellent view of the nerve root canals, whose narrowing plays such an important role in spinal stenosis.

During a CT scan the patient lies on a narrow, adjustable table that moves at a controllable rate through the tunnel-like scanner, which beams low dosage X rays at its target. The angle of the scanner can also be adjusted, thereby increasing the number of planes at which an organ or structure can be x-rayed.

The procedure does not hurt, but it is very lengthy, taking, on average, an hour and a half. Many patients complain that it is difficult to hold still for such a long time, that the "tunnel" makes them feel claustrophobic, and that the noise of the apparatus is "deafening." As for myelography, a dye is sometimes used in conjunction with a CT scan to outline some of the structures that are being x-rayed.

Somato-Sensory Evoked Potentials (SSEP)

Spinal nerves conduct nerve signals differently when chronically compressed than when functioning normally. By measuring the characteristics of the transmitted nerve signal, physicians may be able to localize the nerve that might be responsible for causing a patient's back, leg, neck, or arm pain. The SSEP test thus provides physicians with a neural road map that identifies neurologic deficits. For example, if a patient's arm hurts, the physician can now measure whether the nerve that innervates the right arm is compressed. The SSEP test is often used during spinal surgery to indicate whether a particular operation restores normal nerve transmission. Furthermore, monitoring spinal surgery with SSEP insures that there is no disruption of the nervous system during the operation. The procedure is noninvasive.

Magnetic Resonance Imaging (MRI)

This newer technique combines a magnetic field with radio pulses. It enables physicians to visualize the entire spine and its associated soft tissues, including the spinal cord, spinal nerves, intervertebral disks, fluid, and the size of the bony canals. This procedure does not require X-ray radiation or injection of a dye.

During the procedure the patient lies in a special tunnel-like chamber. The magnetic resonator is programmed to take images of the spine at regular intervals. Like the CT scan, MRI produces images of thin slices of the spine and of the detailed structure of the blood vessels, nerves,tendons, disks, bones, etc. During the procedure, which lasts thirty minutes or more, the patient has to lie very still. Magnetic resonance scans are also used to examine other parts of the body. The procedure, however, cannot be used for patients with magnetic metal implants, such as a pacemaker or the clips used in vascular surgery.

MEDICAL MANAGEMENT

The majority of patients suffering from spinal osteoarthritis do not require surgery. Treatment is divided into managing the acute episode and learning how to live successfully with chronic arthritis of the back. The latter may require learning how to perform certain tasks differently. The site of the osteoarthritic lesions influences the prescribed treatment.

Basically, medical management of degenerative back problems is typical of that used for other joints affected by osteoarthritis.

Pain relief relies on aspirin, Tylenol, and the newer NSAIDs discussed in Chapter 4. Occasionally physicians prescribe a stronger analgesic such as Darvon, or a tranquilizer such as Valium.

Since the back is weight-bearing, rest is particularly important. Persons suffering severe back pain were once ordered to bed for weeks at a time. Since bed rest is debilitating and promotes a weakening of the muscles, most physicians now try to limit total rest to one or two days. The most relaxing sleeping and resting position, as far as the back is concerned, is lying on the side or on the back with knees bent.

Osteoarthritis of the Lower Back

Braces and lumbar corsets, with or without metal stays, are used to reduce motion of the back. The effect of corsets is variable. Some people feel good when they put on a corset; others feel good when they take it off. A patient's response to a corset may provide some information about the nature of the underlying lesion. The prolonged wearing of corsets or other external supports is inadvisable, however, because their use weakens the muscles surrounding the spine.

Other helpful measures for the relief of osteoarthritis of the lower back include

- sleeping on a firm, nonsagging mattress
- sitting in a good chair with armrests and an adjustable high backrest
- sitting straight, with feet flat on the floor and knees at a 90° angle (if necessary, use a footstool or platform for the feet)
- using of one of the many available back support pillows—in the car, at the office, and even at a restaurant
- lying down for thirty to sixty minutes once or twice a day
- avoiding additional back stress (lifting, bending, carrying heavy packages, and bending knees)
- minimizing prolonged immobility (people with desk jobs should get up at least once an hour and walk around)
- Switching chairs during the day (some people love the Scandinavian backless chairs in which some of the weight is transferred from the back to the knees, when "sitting" in this manner, the back posture is close to the standing position)
- putting one foot on a step stool when standing still for a long time
- working at a lectern when possible

Osteoarthritis of the Neck

Proper alignment of the head and neck and reduced motion often alleviate pain. Relief can be obtained by

- sleeping on a cervical pillow or wearing a soft cervical collar at night and even during the day
- wearing a collar if discomfort is severe (to promote strengthening of the neck muscles, the wearing of hard collars is limited usually to two or three weeks)

- using a chair with a headrest
- avoiding reading or watching television when lying down
- avoiding some sports and activities—such as swimming, tennis, or driving—that require frequent turning of the head (swimmers should experiment with style: the backstroke, during which the neck rests on the water, does not stress the neck; the breaststroke—which only involves raising and lowering of the head—may be fine, whereas the crawl—which involves turning the head—may not; drivers should rely on side mirrors, and when on highways, change lanes as infrequently as possible)

Other measures include the following:

Traction: This can be helpful in the short run.

Cold: Initially, during the acute episode, cold compresses are helpful.

Heat: Heat is more effective for chronic pain. For details concerning heat and cold, see Chapter 6, "Rehabilitation and Pain Management."

Exercise: Although bed rest may be helpful in relieving pain and discomfort, it is obviously not a permanent solution. Once the acute symptoms have disappeared, a carefully planned return to normal activity is important. To begin with, the exercises (prescribed by the treating physician and preferably done under the supervision of a physical therapist) will emphasize back movements that are not painful. (See also Chapter 5 for more on exercise and physical therapy.)

Strengthening exercises are introduced thereafter. Many back exercises concentrate on the abdominal muscles, but the strengthening of other back muscles is just as important.

As usual, the formal exercises are supplemented with activities to improve overall fitness. Exercises performed in water, which relieves the spine of much weight, are excellent. Suitable activities are walking in chest-high water or in deep water with an AquaJogger (a large flotation belt available in sports stores or specialized catalogs), aqua calisthenics, and swimming. (See Chapter 5 for details.)

Epidural injection: Corticosteroid injections are occasionally used for the treatment of spinal osteoarthritis. A degenerating disk and/or a narrowed nerve canal may pinch a specific spinal nerve, causing it to become irritated and swollen. Injecting a mixture of steroids and anesthetics into the area surrounding the nerve may help it to shrink.

Epidural injections are a temporary measure that may enable patient and physician to delay surgery for quite some time.

Upper/Lower Back School

As discussed, many back problems are related to poor posture. Chapter 5 reviews healthy ways of sitting, sleeping, and lifting. Back problems are so common that many employers, hospitals, Y's, and other institutions have organized Back Schools, at which participants are taught how to take care of their back. Most of these programs are helpful and recommended.

Surgery

The decades that witnessed the birth of total joint replacements for hips, knees and shoulders also saw enormous progress in spinal surgery.

In 1963 a French surgeon introduced the use of special screws and rods in back surgery. This enabled surgeons to grip and fix the bones of the spine in such a way that they stayed put long enough for the spine to fuse. Instead of having to wear body casts for months, patients could now walk out of the hospital unfettered. These new techniques arrived in the United States during the 1980s.

Metal implants were not the only developments that permitted spinal surgery to expand. Improved diagnostic techniques, new blood preservation techniques, and better methods of anesthesia also made major contributions.

Opting for Surgery

All these new techniques do not necessarily make it easier to opt for surgery. The decision is a hard one for both the doctor and the patient. Most people are extremely afraid of spinal surgery and decide in favor of it only after a long debate. Even though spinal surgery is now safe, most patients are still cautious about undergoing elective back operations. Since few operations yield a "perfect" back, satisfaction with the outcome is a matter of attitude. When making the decision to have back surgery, ask yourself whether you will be content with a partial improvement. Some patients end up happy because they realize that the surgery enabled them to do many things they could not do before. Others, with as successful an outcome, are dissatisfied because their back is definitely not as good as "new."

Here is a checklist for patients contemplating back surgery (see also Chapter 8, "Should You Have Surgery?"):

- Do you understand the reason for the surgery, as well as what the procedure will or will not do?
- Do you trust your surgeon implicitly?
- Are you convinced that all nonsurgical options have been tried?
- Have you allowed yourself plenty of time for recovery?
- Do you understand that the physical shape that you are in before the surgery will contribute to the speed at which you will recover? (A professional athlete will recover faster from any kind of surgery than someone who spends his day at a computer.)
- Are your expectations realistic?

The Operating Room

Lumbar Fusion

As Sam P. grew older, he developed several medical problems, some aggravated by his smoking habit. A few years ago he developed severe back pain and had back surgery. Then he needed a cardiac bypass. But he still was not well. Several years after his original back surgery, his back pain was again acute.

After an in-depth diagnostic investigation, it was decided that Sam required more extensive surgery: a two-stage posterior and anterior fusion. This morning's surgery would fuse the anterior portion of lumbar vertebrae 2, 3, and 4.

It is 9:00 A.M. In the operating room the doctors, nurses, and technologists are getting ready. Sam is stretched out on his back, breathing peacefully. He is under general anesthesia.

Sam's X rays, prominently displayed on the light box, show a metal rod running along the posterior portion of L2 to L4 (lumbar disks 2 to 4).

In many patients such a posterior fusion might have been enough of a repair. The detailed diagnostic studies, however, had revealed that Sam's anterior lumbar disks were deteriorating rapidly and that in the affected part of the spine the bone appeared very weak. His surgeon believed that within a matter of months the metal rod would break down and Sam would again have pain. Rather than wait, his doctor decided to remove the anterior portion of disks L 2–3 and 3–4. Sam was a heavy cigarette smoker. Smoking impairs blood circulation, and this interferes with the healing process. In smokers, some back surgeons prefer to add an anterior to a posterior fusion.

The surgical approach to the spine is either anterior (from the front) or posterior (from the back). The space left by the removed disks in the anterior setting is always filled with bone removed from the patient's own body or obtained from an allograft (see below). Bone is often taken from the iliac crest (the upper portion of the pelvic bone).

Since lumbar vertebral disks are quite thick, the use of bone to fill the gap is often insufficient. Metal rods are often used when the disks are removed from the posterior portion of the spine. These rods are fastened to the vertebrae with screws.

Preparing Sam for the actual surgery took more than an hour. One of the residents shaved Sam's abdomen and scrubbed it with Betadine—a strong disinfectant solution. Then he was positioned so that he was slightly turned onto his side, his buttocks and upper back firmly resting against a clamped bolster, his legs gently crossed. The assistant surgeons draped the patient with green sheets, leaving only a small area of flesh exposed.

The sheets hid the tubes that drained away Sam's body fluids. A complex centrifuge is readied to receive the blood the patient will lose during the operation. Later, this cleaned blood will be reinfused.

Two separate systems supply Sam P.'s body with heat. The first consists of warm water continuously flowing through a blanket. Another, called the Bair Hugger, circulates warm air through a second set of hidden tubes.

Electrodes taped to Sam's feet, ankles, and head lead to the somatosensory evoked potential machine. Should Sam's nerve transmission become abnormal during the surgery, the SSEP technologist will immediately alert the surgeon. According to the technologist, Sam's responses are slow—indicating that he had some previous peripheral nerve damage—but consistent. No trouble is expected.

Three nurses heap boxes of surgical instruments onto movable carts and wheel these close to the patient. The doctor checks on the allograft, a piece of human femoral bone obtained from a bone bank. Special treatment has made it free of communicable diseases. The allograft will be used after the disks have been removed from Sam's spine.

Now the surgeons open the abdominal wall and create a large opening. Eventually the spine appears. The surgeons insert two metal pins that demarcate the regions of the spine in need of repair.

Soon the head surgeon, wearing a special headlight, is ready to remove the anterior portion of disks L2–3 and L3–4. He, his two assistants, and the operating room nurses work quickly, removing pieces of Sam's disks from deep within the cavity. These pieces are placed in sterile Petri dishes and rushed to the orthopedic research laboratory, where they may be used to probe into the causes of degenerative joint disease.

Sam is now ready to be put back together. The exposed portion of the lumbar spine is neat and clean. Instead of degenerated disks, there are now two neat spaces between anterior lumbar vertebrae 2, 3, and 4.

The surgeons now tackle the three-inch allograft. After extracting it from many sterile wrappings, the surgeon slices it to a thickness that fits exactly into the space left after the removal of the disks. The prepared implant now looks surprisingly like the round bone of a shoulder lamb chop.

One of the assistant surgeons enlarges the central hole of the allograft and packs it with slivers of Sam's own iliac crest bone. Since bone regenerates itself, the cells of these bone chips should proliferate and anchor the allograft to the spine. Before continuing with the operation, the surgeon makes sure that the allograft fits.

The allograft to replace the second disk is packed with bone chips, tried for size, and finally slid into place. Sam's exposed lumbar spine looks nice and neat.

Sam's blood vessels, organs, and layers of muscle, fat, and skin are repositioned. The operation is over. The SSEP technologist disconnects the electrodes; the anesthesiologist ceases the administration of anesthetics. Sam, remaining tethered to vital monitoring devices, will wake up in the recovery room.

Spinal Stenosis

During a museum visit, Gail B.'s right leg started to hurt so badly that she kept sitting down. Once back at home she consulted her internist, who determined quickly that Gail did not suffer from phlebitis. An X ray showed no dramatic changes. Gail ignored the pain as best as she could and kept working. But the pain persisted. Eventually it was so bad that when she woke up in the morning her right leg tingled and she could hardly walk.

A CT scan showed that Gail's suffered from spinal stenosis at L4 and L5 (lumbar disks 4 and 5). Stenosis means the abnormal narrowing of a passage. In the case of the spine, it signifies that the passageway through which the nerve roots exit from the spinal canal has narrowed (the cause is often OA). Bone now presses on the nerves, causing pain and dysfunction.

In the hope of alleviating Gail's condition, a physiatrist prescribed exercises, heat, massage, and other modalities, but nothing helped. Two years after she first became aware of her problem, Gail opted for surgery.

Bony overgrowth had narrowed the nerve canal at L4 and L5 and compressed the nerve root as it exited from the spinal sac. Restoration of normal function required the surgical widening of the nerve channel. The term for this type of surgery is *decompression.*

Sometimes decompression surgery simply involves a widening of the nerve root exit. This may involve removing part or all of the *laminae,* or bony arches that form the spinal canal. This operation is called a *laminectomy.*

Often, however, the bony overgrowth is extensive and involves adjoining bones. The resulting alterations of the spinal architecture may affect the intervertebral disks. Then, as in Gail's case, decompression surgery is combined with a fusion.

Since the quality of Gail's vertebrae was good—there was no evidence of osteoporosis—she did not need a metal rod stabilizing her spine. Bone was used to fuse the bones together after excision of part of the disks. After eight days in the hospital, Gail returned home to be cared for by her loving family.

Gail's surgery was a success. Her recovery, however, was slow. In the beginning she was housebound. Finally, after eight weeks, she was allowed to ride in a car. She was cautioned to enter the car carefully without twisting her back. She would sit down on the seat, feet outside the car, then swing over both legs together. This turning motion avoids twisting the back. Gail got out of the car the same way: turning until both legs were outside the car, then standing up. To get in and out of the shower, she sat on the rim of the bathtub, swinging both legs into the tub. It would be months until she was allowed to take a sit-down bath.

While in the hospital, Gail was fitted with a brace that went from under her breast to her hip bone. At first she had to wear the brace around the clock; then only at night. She had hoped that she would wear the brace for three months only. It turned out that it took six months for her fusion to heal sufficiently so that she could walk about safely without the brace. Even after, that there were times when her back acted up and the surgeon advised her to wear her brace for a couple of months.

Within a year Gail's lumbar spine had mended, but then the doctor diagnosed osteoarthritis in her cervical spine. She manages this new problem with physical therapy and swimming the backstroke for twenty minutes three times a week. Gail is fine. She travels, goes to museums, and baby-sits for her four grandchildren.

◆ CHAPTER ◆

12

The Shoulder

Harry F. sighed. His body was out of shape. He used to be very athletic, excelling at golf, tennis, swimming, and skiing. Then each of these activities began to bother his left shoulder, and he abandoned them one by one. Through the years he had also been a sound sleeper, but no more. No matter how carefully he arranged himself in bed, he always ended up rolling onto his arthritic shoulder. Instantly he would wake up with a painful start. It was time to go back to see his orthopedist.

Anatomy of the Shoulder

Many surgeons and physical therapists love the shoulder because of its versatility, complexity, and mobility. The shoulder's mobility and almost global range of motion allow the hand to position itself anywhere on the body. The shoulder is crucial to every major activity of the upper extremity. It is equally comfortable enabling the arm and hand to wield a sledge hammer or deliver a tender caress.

In most people the shoulder is the widest part of the body. Both literally and figuratively it "bears our burdens." Its minimal bony support, however, makes it inherently unstable. Therefore, the shoulder stability depends on ligaments and muscle tissue.

Bony Structure

Three bones meet at the shoulder:

- The *humerus,* or upper arm bone, whose head is almost a perfect sphere.
- The *shoulder blade,* or *scapula,* a large, flat, triangular bone whose upper edge protrudes from the back. The scapula serves as an anchor for the muscles of the upper limbs. These muscles attach to several bones and bony processes: the *glenoid,* the *coracoid,* and the *spine of the scapula,* a ridge which runs across the posterior surface of the scapula ending in the *acromion,* or tip of the scapula. At its upper outer edge, below the acromion, the scapula forms the *glenoid fossa* or glenoid cavity, a socketlike depression which fits the head of the humerus.
- The *collarbone,* or *clavicle,* a long slender bone that connects the bony acromion process, located at the outer edge of the shoulder blade, to the chest bone or sternum. If you press your collarbone with your fingers, you can easily feel how it moves as you raise and lower your arm. The outer edge of the clavicle is the *acromial end;* the inner edge is the *sternal end.*

Soft Tissues

Joints

Unlike the hip, the shoulder is actually a conglomerate of four joints. These are sometimes collectively referred to as the *shoulder girdle.*

- The main shoulder joint is the *glenohumeral joint,* which connects the head of the humerus with the shoulder blade. It is a ball-and-socket joint like the hip, except that the socket—the glenoid fossa—is much shallower than the acetabulum, and dislocation ("popping out") of the shoulder occurs rather frequently.

The other two true joints of the shoulder are:

- The *acromioclavicular joint,* which connects the tip of the shoulder blade, or acromial process, with the acromial extremity of the clavicle.

FIGURE 12-1: *The Shoulder*

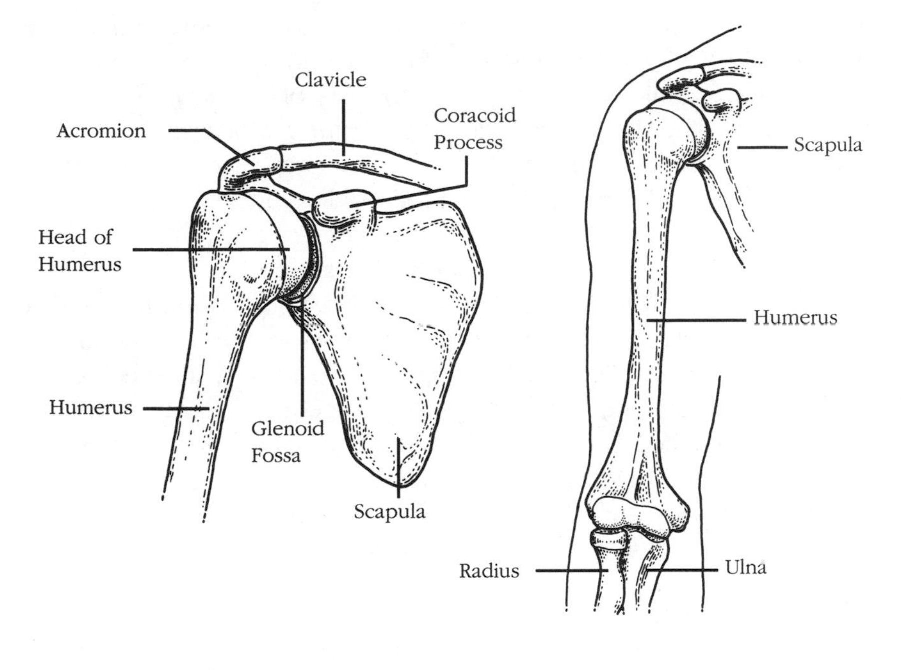

The shoulder or shoulder girdle is a conglomeration of four joints that attach the arm to the trunk. The principal bones involved are the humerus (upper arm bone), the scapula (shoulder blade), and the clavicle (collarbone). The glenohumeral joint, which often develops osteoarthritis, is formed by the upper end of the humerus and the glenoid cavity of the scapula. It is a ball-and-socket joint like the hip, except that the socket—the glenoid fossa—is much shallower than the acetabulum.

- The *sternoclavicular joint,* which connects the sternal extremity of the clavicle with the sternum. Like the gleno-humeral joint, these two joints can develop OA.
- The fourth joint, the *scapulothoracic joint,* attaches the bottom edge of the shoulder blade to the chest or thorax. It is not a true diarthroidal joint and does not develop OA. The scapulothoracic joint enables the lower portion of the scapula to glide over the thorax.

Muscles

Because of its anatomical structure, the stability and strength of the shoulder rests on its deep muscles, tendons, and ligaments.

The fleshy bulk of the shoulder consists of the *scapulothoracic muscles,* including the *trapezius* and the *serratus anterior.* These muscles originate in the chest wall, back, and neck. They stabilize the shoulder blade and provide the entire shoulder with power.

The *deltoid* muscle, which forms the rounded cap of the shoulder, provides strength and leverage to the upper arm.

Four smaller muscles, the *subscapularis, supraspinatus, infraspinatus, and teres minor,* form a perfect envelope around the glenohumeral joint. Collectively these muscles are known as the *rotator cuff,* which, by holding the head of the humerus in its proper place, is essential to shoulder stability. The rotator cuff also enables the shoulder to rotate in the desired direction.

Other muscles contributing to shoulder and upper arm motion include the *pectoralis major* and the *biceps.*

Other Structures

For stability, motion, and smooth function the shoulder depends on numerous tendons, ligaments, and bursae—all of which can become injured, inflamed or diseased. The synovial lining of the joint capsule of the glenohumeral joint can, for instance, become thickened and inflamed. The characteristic "frozen shoulder syndrome" can have a variety of causes. The condition is treated with analgesics, anti-inflammatories, and, if necessary, corticosteroid injections.

Osteoarthritis of the Shoulder

Osteoarthritis of the shoulder is fairly common, often affecting active people. The cause is unknown. Harry F. attributes his OA to trauma he experienced while he was in the Navy during World War II. At the time he repeatedly dislocated his left shoulder. But since his right, uninjured shoulder is also osteoarthritic—though to a lesser extent—trauma cannot be the sole factor in this case.

As always, osteoarthritis develops slowly. The first symptom is pain that occurs only after physical activity or prolonged immobility. When the osteoarthritis is more advanced, patients may come to the doctor complaining that they cannot sleep on the side of the affected shoulder, or that their shoulder is stiff and painful when they wake. Gradually there is loss of function and mobility. Many patients complain of pain experienced while combing their hair, reaching for an object on a high shelf, and washing the armpit on the opposite side of the body, eventually there is an inability to perform self-care at the toilet.

DIAGNOSIS

Diagnosis is complicated since the shoulder develops many aches and pains, most of them not related to arthritis. One medical textbook lists twenty-three common causes of referred shoulder pain—including heart disease (myocardial insufficiency), pulmonary conditions, gallbladder disease, and ectopic pregnancy. Much more closely related to the shoulder are disorders involving the cervical region of the spine (the neck). Indeed, the shoulder and the neck are so closely interrelated that the two often have to be dealt with as a unit.

In addition to these nonshoulder problems, the shoulder itself can develop a host of nonarthritic disorders—including bursitis, tendinitis, dislocations, and tearing of one of the muscles.

Fortunately, a skilled physician can eliminate many of these possible diagnoses by carefully examining the shoulder and taking a detailed medical history. The physician will take great care in examining the patient's movement from both the front and the back. A thorough examination establishes the range of motion of the shoulder (active, passive, flexion-extension, external and internal rotation, elevation, etc.) Key indications are the presence of trigger sites at which the pain can be elicited; swelling, redness, or warmth; and tenderness and pain upon motion.

A skilled observer also notices immediately how patients with shoulder pain move. They attempt to protect their shoulder and may exhibit slight postural changes. They may, for instance, walk with bent elbows to reduce shoulder stress, turn their hurting shoulder inward, or hunch up their healthy shoulder and tilt their neck towards it. They avoid using the hurting arm as much as possible.

During the medical interview the doctor will ask you many questions about pain and stiffness patterns, such as the following:

- Is the pain more pronounced in the morning after getting up? In the evening? When using the arm? After exercise?
- Does your work or recreational activity involve much reaching above your head? For instance, house painting, tennis, shelving books, and putting away groceries may all strain the shoulder.
- Do you recall any incident that might have damaged your shoulder, such as a fall or car accident?

An X ray confirms a diagnosis. Early osteoarthritis is marked by joint space narrowing. As the disease progresses, the smooth hyaline surface is pitted, becoming increasingly uneven. More advanced disease is characterized by osteophyte formation. Eventually the shoulder cartilage wears out, and bone rubs on bone. (See Chapter 3 for more on the development of OA.)

Medical Treatment

Drug Therapy

Aspirin, newer NSAIDs, and acetaminophen are the drugs of choice for osteoarthritis of the shoulder (see Chapter 4). Local steroid injections (see Chapter 13) often offer only temporary relief, usually not lasting more than several weeks.

Joint Protection

The rest-and-exercise dictum is particularly important for the shoulder, because its joint capsule and ligaments have a tendency to thicken so that the joint becomes stiff and even "frozen." Shoulder exercises are a must, but so is rest and joint protection.

During acute shoulder pain it is important to carry your arm in a sling. This assists the healing process. Slings can be bought at a pharmacy or made at home from a large square scarf. Additional stress, such as carrying heavy briefcases or shopping bags, must be avoided. When the shoulder pain originates in the nearby cervical neck, it is often helpful to wear a soft cervical collar, sometimes only while sleeping. By reducing the movement of the cervical vertebrae, such a collar may relieve pain.

Physical Therapy

The shoulder is delicate, and exercises should be carefully prescribed. Since the shoulder "freezes" easily, range-of-motion and stretching exercises are particularly important. (See also Chapter 13 for more on range-of-motion exercises.)

Start the exercises prescribed by your physician by warming up your shoulder with a hot shower, heating pad, or hot water bottle.

The Long Road to Surgery

Harry F. is an expert on medical treatment. He dislocated his shoulder in 1945 while riding a freight train in the Navy. Harry F. sat on the car directly behind the engine. When smoke engulfed him, he jumped from flatbed to flatbed toward the end of the train. Suddenly he missed and fell into an empty oil drum, dislocating his shoulder. The shoulder was put back into place, only to dislocate twice more. When Harry got back to the United States, an orthopedic surgeon repaired the soft tissues of his shoulder.

After a lot of physical therapy, Harry F.'s fixed-up shoulder served him well for more than twenty-five years. Golf was his favorite sport, but he also enjoyed tennis, basketball, and swimming. Then, gradually, his shoulder began to act up. At first it just felt tired after a long round of golf or a long swim. He felt the shoulder "catch" when he played basketball. He had trouble tossing the ball into the air when he served at tennis.

Harry's internist diagnosed osteoarthritis in both shoulders. Harry F. started taking Tylenol and Advil for the pain and had some physical therapy and massages. The internist also referred Harry to an orthopedist specializing in shoulder problems. The specialist advised him that his osteoarthritis had progressed to the point that he should consider reconstructive surgery.

Overall Design of the Total Shoulder Prosthesis

Mild osteoarthritis of the shoulder can often be treated by arthroscopy. As with arthroscopy of the knee, the arthroscope can be used to remove loose bodies and bone spurs, debride or clean the joint, or clean an inflamed synovium. Other shoulder problems often involve soft tissue surgery.

The "total" shoulder, which is the third most frequently performed joint replacement surgery, was developed at Columbia Presbyterian. Compared to other joints, the shoulder prosthesis has had a rather long history. By 1951 a prosthesis for the head of the humerus had been developed by Dr. Charles Neer II. The prosthesis had an umbrellalike head that replaced the head of the humerus, and a metal stem that was inserted into its canal. The shape of the prosthesis allowed much of the normal anatomy and musculature of the shoulder to remain intact. In fact, it enabled the surgeon to cut away only a small portion of the head of the humerus and still achieve success. Holes left in the base of the "umbrella" permitted in-growth of bone.

This prosthesis was used for twenty years with excellent results. After surgery patients were able to return to their prior occupations—including carpentry, farming, and other heavy labor—without any loosening of their prostheses. The operation was, however, successful only for patients in whom the glenoid portion of the shoulder joint was normal or only minimally affected by arthritis.

Stimulated by the advent of the total hip joint replacement, doctors decided to develop a total prosthesis to repair shoulders in which both sides of the glenohumeral joint were damaged by the arthritic process.

In 1973, doctors at Columbia Presbyterian developed a prosthesis that had a conforming surface (i.e., it fit the anatomic structure) and was minimally constraining (limiting). Once in place the humeral head and glenoid portion closely approximate the normal anatomy of the shoulder. This Neer II system became the most popular "total shoulder" and is today used the world over.

Total shoulder replacement has a success rate of over 95 percent. The operation is usually done under regional anesthesia. Harry F. was a little bit squeamish about being awake during the three-and-a-half-hour operation, but his anesthesiologist told him that he "would not remember a thing."

Like Dorothy O., our knee patient, Harry F. thought that he would check into the hospital the day before the surgery. "No," he was told, "come at eleven A.M., the day of the operation." When he arrived he was told to hurry, because surgery was at noon. Harry F. was shown to a locker room, where he took off his street clothes and, refusing a wheelchair, walked into the operating theater. As soon as he was settled on the table, he received a sodium pentothal anesthesia; the rest, to him, is indeed a blur. He woke in the operating room and felt the surgeon removing the tape pasted to his back. The few hours he spent in the recovery room were uneventful. That night he slept happily in a beautiful room overlooking the Hudson River. (For details of shoulder surgery, see below.)

Rehabilitation

A physical therapist came the next day, moved his arm, and initiated gentle pendulum exercises the day after that. (Pendulum exercises involve swinging the arm back and forth.)

At first Harry F. wore a sling all the time, but on the fourth day after the operation, the surgeon said that he could take the sling off when sitting in bed or on a chair. When around and about, Harry F. will wear the sling for several weeks until the shoulder is safely set.

Five days after the surgery Harry F. went home. For one week he went every day to out-patient physical therapy; then he, too, was on his own. As a matter of fact, he made plans to move to Vermont. By the following summer he should be able to swim, golf, and play tennis.

Complications

As in all total joint replacement surgery, complications can occur after a total shoulder is done. These may involve infection, dislocation, or loosening or tearing of the rotator cuff muscles. The complication rate, however, is low. In one study there were only four infections among 1,168 cases. As with hip and knee complications, treatment involves cleaning or removal of the prosthesis and long-term antibiotic therapy.

Surgical Replacement of the Head of the Humerus

Like Harry, Vera H. had had shoulder pain for more than twenty years. By now her right shoulder was almost totally useless. Physical therapy, NSAIDS, and periodic corticosteroid injections no longer provided relief, and Vera's internist referred her to an orthopedist specializing in the shoulder. He confirmed that the seventy-two-year-old patient suffered from advanced osteoarthritis of the shoulder, and after much deliberation he decided that Vera was medically fit to undergo total shoulder replacement.

◆ ◆ ◆ ◆ ◆ ◆ ◆

Like Harry, Vera arrives at the hospital the morning of her surgery. She, however, insists on having total anesthesia and is heavily sedated when attendants position her on the operating room table.

Two anesthesiologists administer the general anesthesia, and soon Vera breathes regularly and deeply. The surgeons and his assistants arrange Vera in a semisitting position and cover her entire body with blue sheets. Only her right arm and shoulder protrude.

Vera's X rays are displayed on the light box. The joint space between the humerus and the glenoid cavity is almost gone, and osteoarthritis pits the head of the humerus.

The surgeons shave off a few remaining hairs on Vera's arm, scrub it lengthily with Betadine antiseptic solution, and paste a sterile plastic sheet over her shoulder and upper arm. Then her lower arm is covered with a sleeve. Only a square foot of plastic-covered flesh is visible.

The head surgeon makes a 12-centimeter incision into the skin that covers the shoulder. He works extremely carefully and cautiously so as to avoid damaging any of Vera's muscles, nerves, tendons, and blood vessels. The shoulder joint is complex, with many important soft tissue structures that must be preserved to allow optimum function. During the surgery there is indeed minimal blood loss as the surgeon retracts the major shoulder muscles and approaches the shoulder joint.

Nevertheless, the surgeon is not pleased. "Look," he tells his assistants, "she has a torn rotator cuff, which we must repair as well as we can." Fortunately, a direct inspection of the glenoid cavity reveals that it is relatively free of osteoarthritis.

Plans for the surgery are instantly changed. Instead of a "total shoulder," the surgeon will simply replace the head of the humerus, which is severely destroyed by osteoarthritis. Large osteophytes ring its lower edge. These are removed with care. Between the muscle tissues are white deposits, the remains of old corticosteroid injections. These too are removed.

Using a two-dimensional model, the surgeon measures the humerus for size before proceeding. "A size twenty-two will do," he tells his assistants. After some more measurements the surgeon cuts off the head of the humerus with an oscillating saw at a 45° angle. The removed bone is placed in a small dish and sent to the laboratory.

Once he is satisfied with the angle of the cut, the surgeon prepares the humeral canal to receive the appropriate-size stem. A small stem will do for this small-boned woman. The fit is tight and the stem will not be cemented in place. As with hip replacements, whether or not to cement a prosthesis in place is the subject of much scientific debate.

Even though she will not be implanted with a total shoulder, the surgeon expects Vera to be pain-free, with good function.

If Vera had needed the glenoid portion of the total shoulder prosthesis in addition to the humeral part, thc surgeon would have reamed out the glenoid cavity. Then he would have drilled a hole into its center and cemented the high density glenoid plateau in place.

Once he is convinced that the new head of the humerus articulates freely with the glenoid cavity, the surgeon repairs the rotator cuff. Then he carefully repositions the muscle tissue and closes the skin. The operation is over. Vera's arm is bandaged and fastened to a large splint. The anesthesiologists discontinue the anesthesia. Vera is transferred to the recovery room, and a few hours later she'll wake up in her room.

◆ CHAPTER ◆

13

The Hand, Wrist, and Elbow

The hand, like the brain, is characteristically human, the one carrying out the commands of the other. Figures of speech using the hand are abstract. Being helpful is "lending a hand"; being fair is being "even-handed"; arguments are carefully evaluated "on the one hand or on the other"; and when "your left hand does not know what your right one is doing," you are in trouble.

Our hands are complex and versatile. They can deliver a powerful punch, thread the eye of a needle, or play a violin. Hands also function as sensors, feeding the brain essential information about shape, texture, size, and distance.

Anatomy of the Hand

The Bones and Joints of the Hand

When first consulting a hand specialist, you may be confused by his or her referring to metacarpophalangeal, proximal interphalangeal, or distal interphalangeal joints. A look at Figure 13-1 clarifies the matter.

Each hand and wrist together consist of twenty-seven separate bones, all connected by cartilage, tendons, and muscles. The wrist consists of eight small, round bones collectively called the *carpus.* These bones function like a ball bearing, facilitating the rotary movements of the wrist. One of the carpal bones at the base of the thumb, the *trapezium,* is of special concern and we will discuss it in detail later.

Each finger ray consists of four elongated bones (the thumb has only three). The bones closest to the wrist are called the *metacarpals;* the other three are the *phalanges.* (The word *phalanx* comes from the Greek and means "line or array of soldiers.") To distinguish the phalanges from one another they are called, from the palms out, the *proximal phalanx,* the *middle phalanx,* and the *distal phalanx.*

To figure out which joint is which, remember that physicians and anatomists designate any bone, bone end, or joint close to the center of the body as *proximal,* and any more distant part *distal.* Joints are named after the two bones they connect. In the case of the hand we have

- the carpal-metacarpal joints (CMC)
- the metacarpal-phalangeal joints (MCP)
- the proximal interphalangeal joints (PIP)
- the distal interphalangeal joints (DIP)

The joint at the base of the thumb—which often is a target of osteoarthritis—is called the trapezio-metacarpal (TM) joint.

The joints of the four long fingers have a characteristic tongue-and-groove shape that provides the highly exposed finger joints with stability.

Muscles and Hand Movements

The intricate motion of the entire hand is dependent on muscles that originate in the forearm and in the hand itself. The muscles originating in the forearm are called the *extrinsic muscles;* those that originate in the hand itself are the *intrinsic muscles.*

The thumb is powered by eight separate muscles and tendons that, together with its unique saddle-shaped joint, make it extremely mobile and versatile. The thumb can rotate and move back and forth and from side to side. The wrist rotates and bends. Each finger flexes (bends) more than ninety degrees, extends (straightens), and abducts (opens and closes sideways). The muscles of the hand are mainly located on the palm side, forming little cushions and creases.

The skin that covers the hand is highly specialized: that covering the palm is tough, allowing the hand to grab heavy objects; the skin covering the top of the hand is loose-fitting, giving the joints plenty of

FIGURE 13-1: *The Hand*

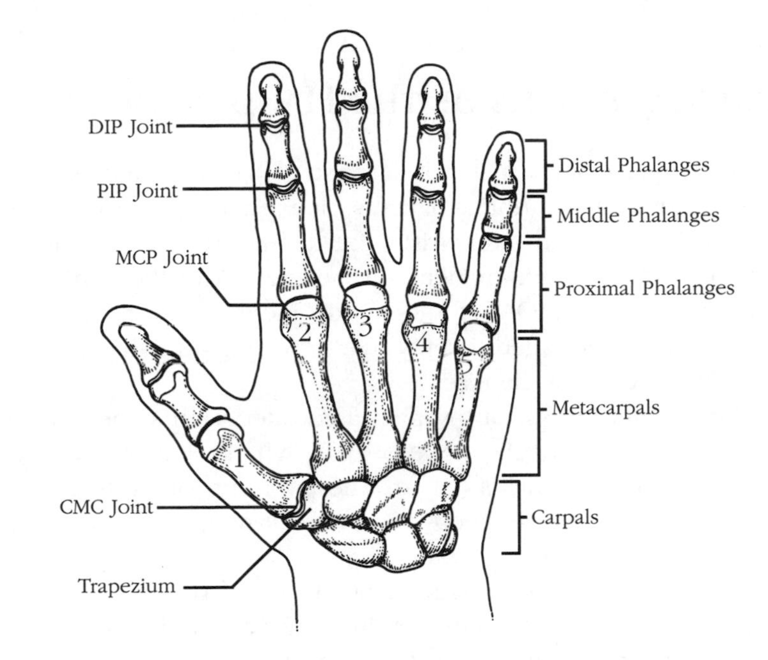

The hand consists of the carpus (wrist) and five rays terminating in the fingers. The eight small bones of the wrist are connected by strong ligaments. Note the trapezium, which articulates with the base of the thumb.

The five elongated metacarpal bones form the palm of the hand. The remaining bones of the hand, fourteen in all, are called the phalanges. Each of the four fingers has three—from the palm outwards, they are the proximal, middle, and distal phalanx. The thumb has only two phalanges.

The tongue-and-groove joints of the hand are named after the bones they connect:

- The carpal-metacarpal joints (CMC)
- The metacarpal-phalangeal joints (MCP)
- The proximal interphalangeal joints (PIP)
- The distal interphalangeal joints (DIP)

The joint at the base of the thumb, discussed in this chapter, is the trapeziometacarpal joint (TM).

space to bend and extend. This slack is necessary to allow for the extra space required when making a fist or grasping.

Osteoarthritis of the Hand

With its many joints, it is not surprising that the hand is a target of osteoarthritis. Of all arthritis patients, one quarter have significant problems with their hands and wrists. Put differently, approximately 8 percent of all adults have moderate to severe OA of the hands and feet. The prevalence of OA of the hands increases with age. Some 85 percent of persons aged seventy-five to seventy-nine have some radiographic evidence of the disease.

One might think that the pain associated with something as small as a finger joint is negligible, especially when compared with as large a joint as the hip. This is not so. The pain in a single finger joint can be so intense that it can keep you awake at night and render the entire hand virtually useless.

The very good news is that the hands of patients suffering from osteoarthritis are rarely as twisted and gnarled as those of patients suffering from the inflammatory forms of arthritis. Many patients, especially women, however, find that with aging their fingers thicken and become stiff.

Osteoarthritis of the hand takes years to develop. Typically the first symptom is stiffness, followed by pain and/or instability.

The development of osteoarthritis in the finger joints is similar to that observed elsewhere. Early overt symptoms are morning stiffness, soreness at the base of the thumb, and a weakened pinch. The joints crepitate (crackle) when moved. The cartilage deteriorates gradually. There is minor inflammation of the synovium, the thin membrane lining the joint capsule—probably triggered by an attempt by the body to clear away the cartilage debris. The underlying denuded bone may respond by forming new bone, which appears as a typically enlarged joint. Lubrication and motion are impaired. Eventually the entire joint malfunctions.

Heberden's Nodes

One form of osteoarthritis that definitely is inherited is the formation of bony knobs on the fingers. Here is how William Heberden, a British physician, mused upon them 250 years ago:

> *What are those little hard knobs, about the size of a small pea, which are frequently seen upon the fingers, particularly a little below the top, near the joint? They have no connection to the gout, being found in persons who never had it. They continue for life; and being hardly ever attended with pain, or disposed to become sores, are rather unsightly, than inconvenient, though they must be some little hindrance to the free use of the fingers.*

William Heberden (1710–1801), in Commentary on the History and Cure of Diseases.

These knobs, now called Heberden's nodes, are a frequent manifestation of osteoarthritis in older women. They form on the distal interphalangeal (DIP) joint. As Heberden stated so long ago, they are more unsightly than disabling. Occasionally fluid-filled cysts occur in conjunction with Heberden's nodes. Effective surgical removal of these so-called "mucous cysts" requires the simultaneous excision of the Heberden's node.

Bouchard's Nodes

Knobs can also form on the proximal interphalangeal (PIP) joint. These nodes are called Bouchard's nodes.

Osteoarthritis of the Trapezio-Metacarpal Joint

Osteoarthritis of the joint at the base of the thumb occurs frequently in older women. Its cause is unclear, but its effect can be rather debilitating. Pain is the first symptom, followed by decreased "pinching ability" and finally instability.

When Alice J. consulted an orthopedist, the thumb of her right hand was so painful that she had trouble cooking. She could not peel potatoes, open jars, or turn a key.

Diagnosis

Upon physical examination, the doctor noted that Alice's trapezio-metacarpal (TM) joint at the base of the thumb was knobby, tender, and weak. An X ray showed that the cartilage was gone, the joint space had narrowed, and bone was rubbing on bone.

MEDICAL TREATMENT

The orthopedist prescribed a splint and NSAIDs, and sent his patient to a hand therapist. Alice J. improved, but not enough.

So her doctor injected Alice's TM joint with corticosteroids, hoping that this medication would suppress her pain and inflammation enough to permit recovery of function.

Intra-Articular Steroid Injections

Corticosteroids, like cortisone or prednisone, are powerful anti-inflammatory drugs sometimes used for rheumatoid arthritis and other in-flammatory forms of the disease. When taken by mouth for prolonged periods of time, these drugs are effective, but may have any number of serious side effects—including (but not limited to) weight gain, hyperglycemia, edema, ulcers, and cataracts. Systemic corticosteroids (taken orally and affecting the entire body) are not used in the treatment of osteoarthritis because here inflammation does not play a major role.

Occasionally corticosteroids are injected into specific osteoarthritic joints. To this end the drugs are formulated so that they remain at the injection site for a number of weeks (this is another use of the slow drug release technique discussed in Chapter 4). By suppressing pain and local inflammation, a depot corticosteroid injection sometimes allows a joint to recover.

The effect of a corticosteroid injection typically lasts four to six weeks or longer. No joint, whether fingers, thumbs, knees, hips, or shoulders, should be injected more than two to three times.

SURGICAL TREATMENT

Alice's pain was somewhat relieved by all these measures, but the respite was temporary, lasting a few weeks only. Her thumb remained painful and useless. She was depressed and disliked wearing her hand splint. Finally, doctor and patient opted for surgical treatment.

Arthroplasty of the Trapezio-Metacarpal Joint

The human hand is a precision instrument, and the surgery it requires is very different from that involving such large anatomical structures as the hip, knee, or back. It is almost always done under local or regional anesthesia, and there is usually no major blood loss. Today hand and foot surgery are usually done as outpatient procedures.

Alice arrived in the operating room on a small stretcher, fully awake. An aide transferred her to the operating room table.

An anesthesiologist injected anesthetic into Alice's arm (regional axillary block). Within twenty minutes her arm lost all sensation. To numb her consciousness Alice also received intravenous Versed, a Valium-like drug.

When she was properly anesthetized, the doctor felt Alice's hand and marked a five-inch line on the wrist with a sterile pen. To halt the blood flow temporarily and operate in a bloodless field, the surgeon fastened a tourniquet around Alice's upper arm. Using a special rubber bandage, the doctor "pushed" the blood remaining in the arm into the general circulation. Blood flow can be interrupted safely for two hours without harming the tissue. Now all was ready, and the doctor cut the skin covering the wrist.

As he pushed back the tissue that covered the carpal bones, the doctor could see that both sides of the trapezio-metacarpal joint were damaged by osteoarthritis. The doctor removed the trapezium, and in so doing excised the worn-out surfaces that caused his patient's pain.

Many of the body's large tendons are found in the lower leg, foot, forearm, and hand. These tendons are colorless, and some are so large that they look like macaroni. The function of these tendons is to effectuate the intricate movements of the hand and the precise motions of the feet. Hand surgery necessitated by arthritis often involves repositioning or repairing some of the tendons damaged by the disease.

The human hand and wrist contain some nonessential tendons, one of which the doctor was going to use to repair Alice's hand. Carefully the surgeon unfastened one of Alice's spare tendons, rolled it up, and inserted it in place of the now-missing carpal bone. Everything was carefully sutured into place. The doctor moved Alice's wrist and fingers to ascertain that the entire hand functioned properly. Because he was able to fill the empty space with Alice's own tissue, his patient did not require any man-made materials. Alice won't miss her tendon, and her wrist will function adequately with seven carpal bones instead of eight.

Before sewing the skin back together, the doctor carefully washed the surgical site with some anti-blood-clotting medication. As soon as he could, the surgeon removed the tourniquet restoring blood flow. "You did just fine," he assured his patient before proceeding to encase her wrist, forearm, and thumb—but not her fingers—in a plaster splint.

No hospital stay was required, and Alice went home the day of her surgery. Unlike hips and knees, hands must be allowed to heal slowly. Alice's wrist was immobilized for two weeks. Then she returned to the hospital. The doctor took off the big splint, decided that it had healed sufficiently, and sent her to hand rehabilitation.

There the occupation therapist fashioned a lighter splint (see below) and showed Alice how to move her repaired joint gently. For another four weeks Alice kept her arm in a sling, but gradually she used it more normally. Full recovery took four to six months.

Alice J. is happy. Her hand is functional and her family once more enjoys her fabulous cooking.

Other Types of Hand Arthroplasty

Alice did not require any prosthesis, but this is not always the case. Today finger joints, mostly destroyed by osteoarthritis or rheumatoid arthritis, are repaired using small, flexible silicone rubber implants. These artificial spacers are inserted in place of the removed, diseased joint. Healthy tendons and muscle tissue are carefully repositioned around the silicone implant. Long-term follow-up in patients with osteoarthritis or rheumatoid arthritis have shown excellent results.

Hand Rehabilitation

The occupational therapist is a rehabilitation specialist who concentrates on finding out what her patients *can do*. Then she helps them increase their performance and often teaches them to do things differently or in a less destructive way. The occupational therapist is especially crucial in the treatment of arthritic hands.

Hand rehabilitation for osteoarthritis combines energy conservation, joint protection techniques, activities of daily living, range-of-motion (ROM) exercises, and—if necessary—splinting. The occupational specialist stresses that, to be successful, rehabilitation entails a team approach that includes the hand surgeon, the occupational therapist, and the rheumatologist. Good communication and cooperation between these professionals optimize the care provided to the patient.

Assessment

To begin with, the occupational therapist (OT) evaluates the function of her patient's hands as well as that of the entire upper arm. She pays close attention to the interaction of the hand and the shoulder. Typical measurements include evaluation of the grip, pinch strength, range of motion, swelling (edema), and sensation.

More important, she has a long list of "activities of daily living" (ADL), which tells her exactly how to focus her therapy. The questions are answered by a simple yes or no. If the patient cannot perform the task independently, the occupational therapist must evaluate how much assistance is required. If necessary and appropriate, she may suggest the use of adaptive equipment, and demonstrate its use. Here is part of the occupational therapist's ADL list:

Dressing: Can you button your shirt (front opening)? Can you button your shirt cuffs? Can you put on an overcoat? A sweater? Can you put on slacks? A skirt? Stockings? Panty hose?

Jewelry: Can you wind a watch? Can you put on a watch? Rings? Bracelets? Tie clasps? Can you manage your hearing aid? Eyeglasses?

Personal Hygiene: Can you manage toothpaste, clean your dentures, shave, cut your toenails, shampoo your hair?

Eating: Can you eat with your fingers, use a fork, knife, spoon, drink from a glass or cup?

Communication: Can you write, handle mail, dial a telephone, use coins in a public telephone, sharpen pencils?

Other: Can you drive, use public transportation, hammer nails, work in the garden, play an instrument, play cards, manage your home, turn on water, light a gas stove, pour hot liquids, use an electric mixer, break an egg, carry pots and pans, retrieve things from the floor, mop the floor, use the vacuum, thread a needle, sew on buttons, knit?

By the time she is through with this evaluation, the occupational therapist has a pretty good idea of what her patient can and cannot do. She structures her therapy accordingly.

Joint Protection

The cornerstone of arthritis therapy is appropriate rest and exercise. For the hands, the first is often provided by splints and by reducing the stress on particular joints.

Splinting

Splinting is one of the oldest methods of resting painful joints. One can imagine a cave man bracing his arthritic leg with a few wooden sticks and some large leaves, then tying the whole thing together with a long vine.

Today splints are made from plastics that are moldable at low temperatures. Polyform, Ezeform, Aquaplast, and other brands are a combination of plastic and rubber. The OT starts out by making a pattern. Then she cuts the plastic to the shape of the pattern, heats the splint in hot water, and molds it to her patient's hand and wrist, leaving enough space to allow the fingers to move freely. The splint is then cooled under running tap water, which "sets" the plastic. Velcro straps complete the splint and allow the patient to take it off at will. This type of splint enables hand patients to use their fingers more easily and without pain.

Joint Conservation (Avoiding Stress)

The small joints of the fingers are among the most exposed and delicate of the body. For anyone suffering from osteoarthritis, it is important to minimize the mechanical stress to which these joints are exposed. Though the hands and fingers are especially vulnerable, the joint protection principles outlined here apply to all joints.

The Arthritis Foundation's *Guide to Independent Living for People with Arthritis* makes countless suggestions on how to modify simple tasks such as opening doors, turning keys, closing zippers, and opening ring-topped cans or milk containers. The *Guide* lists 537 sources that sell adaptive equipment. Items range from the inexpensive—cylinders that slip over eating utensils and handy gadgets to turn control knobs on washers or kitchen stoves—to the more expensive—stairway elevators and window greenhouses for gardening enthusiasts. The *Guide* can be ordered from the Arthritis Foundation. In addition to using special equipment, you can protect your joints by doing the following:

- **Use the largest, strongest joint(s) available to perform a task.** For example, use the palm of your hand instead of your fingers. Hold your coffee mug with both palms of the hand instead of grasping it with your fingers by the handle. Use both hands to pour liquid from a container. Use the heels of your hands to open a window rather than your fingers. Build up the handles of knives, etc. with foam sleeves. When writing, use a pen with a large circumference or type with ten fingers.
- **Avoid muscle fatigue.** For example, do not carry a heavy bag or briefcase for any length of time with the arm extended. Carry loads close to the body using shoulder straps. Wheel groceries in a shopping cart.
- **Rest frequently.** When performing a task requiring sustained joint effort, such as writing or chopping vegetables, take a break and relax your hands.
- **Respect pain.** Modify activities that cause pain.
- **Use your hands and body properly.** For example, avoid using your hands to pull yourself out of a low chair.

Exercises for the Upper Extremity: Hand, Shoulder, Elbow

You also need to build strength in your hands. One does not have to have overt arthritis to profit from hand exercises. Because our hands stiffen as we age, they benefit from regular exercise.

Here are the basic exercises that the occupational therapist prescribes for patients suffering from osteoarthritis of the wrists, elbows, and fingers. Note that some of the exercises are *active* (done without outside assistance), and some are *passive* (done using the other hand to assist the one that is being exercised). The exercises are designed as a home program to maintain passive motion of the joints and muscle tone.

These exercises are used during nonsurgical treatment of the hands. Orthopedic surgeons are very strict about when to start exercising, what exercises to do, and how often to do each exercise. Once or twice a day, repeating each exercise five to ten times, is usual. It is in your best interest to follow the instructions carefully. Hand exercises are highly individualized. Initially they focus on reestablishing the range of motion of the hand; then they emphasize building up strength.

Hand Exercises

1. To maintain or improve joint mobility begin by bringing each joint of the arm through its full range or motion.
2. Soak your hand in a basin of warm water for *twenty minutes.* While soaking, open and close fingers fifteen to twenty times and move wrists back and forth. Patients with very painful joints may precede the exercises by using a paraffin bath (see Heat, below).
3. Massage your hand with lotion, rubbing from your fingertips down past your wrist. Squeeze down each finger individually.

Shoulder Exercises

Raise arms up to chest level with palms down. Open arms out to sides. Turn palms up, and raise arms overhead. Return out to sides, rotate palms down, and bring arms back to chest level in front. Relax as you lower your arms.

Elbow Exercises

1. Straighten elbows and then bend completely.
2. With elbows bent 90° and tucked at sides of body, rotate palms up and down. If your motion is limited, assist with your other hand by grasping the wrist and twisting your palm up and down.
3. Let your hands hang over the arms of a chair. Keeping the fingers relaxed, raise and lower your wrists as much as possible in each direction. If this motion is limited, use your other hand to assist: place hand on top of other hand and push down. Then place hand under palm and push up.

4. Same position as number 7 except forearm is resting on its side. Push wrist down towards your little finger and then raise it up towards your thumb. If this motion is limited, push wrist down using your other hand to assist, and raise it up pushing from underneath.
5. With elbows on a table make tight fists, placing your thumb over your other fingers. Then open as wide as you can. Then, using your other hand to assist, curl each finger down into your palm and straighten each finger up stretching it back.
6. Keeping your fingers straight, spread them apart and bring them together.
7. Resting your hand on its side on the table, bring your thumb down to the table, then out to the side and then up. Then circle in the other direction.
8. Touch your thumb to each fingertip making nice round circles.

Heat

Many persons suffering from arthritis of the hands benefit from dipping their hands into warm—not hot—molten paraffin. After patients remove their hand from the paraffin bath, the wax solidifies, forming a tight glove that slowly gives off heat as it cools. Prolong the cooling-off process by inserting your paraffined hand into a plastic bag. Today small paraffin baths for home use can be ordered from Grimm Box, 2143 Marietta, OH 45750 (1-800-223-5395).

Depending on the model, the small electrically-heated bath costs between $140 and $180. The cost of this bath may be reimbursable by Medicare and some other insurance policies.

Osteoarthritis of the Wrist

Osteoarthritis of the wrist is rather common. The condition most often follows traumatic injury. The arthritis is treated in the usual manner, with rest, splinting, NSAIDs, and gentle exercises.

If these measures fail, and the wrist remains painful and unstable, surgery is sometimes indicated. As we have seen, the wrist consists of eight little bones. Sometimes the arthritis is limited to a few bones which then can be selectively fused, thereby preserving good motion in the remaining parts of the joint.

When the arthritis is severe, the entire wrist may require fusion. A fused wrist is strong and serviceable.

THE ELBOW

The elbow permits the arm to flex and allows the hand to carry food to the mouth. It is a well-engineered, tight joint, poorly cushioned and highly exposed.

Like the leg, the upper extremity consists of three bones: the *humerus,* the upper arm bone; the *ulna,* the larger of the two forearm bones; and the *radius,* the smaller of the two forearm bones, which runs parallel to the ulna.

The elbow, which connects the three bones, is really two joints in one. The "true" elbow joint is a hinge that connects the humerus and the ulna, permitting the forearm and hand to move up and down. The other, smaller joint, connecting the head of the radius and the ulna, allows the forearm to twist and turn almost 180° without moving the upper arm. Both joints are enclosed into one single joint capsule.

At its lower end the humerus widens into a pitchfork-shaped structure. Each tine of the fork terminates in an *epicondyle* (bony outgrowth), to which most of the muscles, ligaments, and tendons of the upper and lower arm are attached. Injury and overuse often cause inflammation of these tendons; this is known as tendinitis. Tennis elbow and golfer's elbow are types of tendinitis that run along the outer and inner epicondyles respectively. The two epicondyles are separated by a deep groove.

The lower end of the humerus has two articular surfaces: the *trochlea,* which is pulley-shaped, and the *capitelum,* which is spherical. These surfaces articulate with the forearm. The *trochlear notch of the ulna* articulates with the trochlea, and the cupped (concave) head of the radius fits the rounded shape of the capitulum.

At its upper end the ulna terminates in a sharp bony angular structure, the *olecranon,* which is the part commonly known as the "elbow." The olecranon is cushioned by a large bursa, the olecranon bursa, which occasionally becomes inflamed.

Osteoarthritis of the Elbow

Primary osteoarthritis of the elbow is rare. When present it occurs more frequently in men than in women. Patients may have a history of heavy arm use, such as weight lifters, pitchers, and other athletes who throw objects. Secondary osteoarthritis, which develops at the site of an old fracture or injury, also occurs. Pain, impaired mobility, and joint space narrowing are early symptoms of osteoarthritis of the elbow. Later stages are characterized by osteophytes. Sometimes elbow pain is due to a loose piece of cartilage or bone that can be removed by arthroscopy.

Medical Treatment

Medical treatment of osteoarthritis of the elbow includes aspirin, Tylenol, and the newer NSAIDs. Applied heat or ice often relieves pain. Rest is important. Hinged splints, which allow active motion, may prove helpful, as may splints worn during the night. It is important to avoid stressing the joint—don't carry groceries, briefcases, or suitcases. As always, range-of-motion and strengthening exercises are important. To mitigate pain and inflammation, the elbow joint is sometimes injected with corticosteroids (see above).

Surgical Treatment

Unlike the wrist, fusion of an arthritic elbow is debilitating because it interferes with function. There simply isn't a single best position in which this joint can be fused.

Developing a total elbow prosthesis has been rather difficult, mostly because the joint is so very exposed and is not cushioned by muscle tissue. Three different prosthetic designs are available: constrained (hinged), semiconstrained, and nonconstrained. As in the case of the knee, constrained prostheses were associated with a high failure rate, and today these devices have largely been abandoned. Results with loose semiconstrained prostheses are more promising. Fortunately, the operation is infrequently needed for patients suffering from osteoarthritis of the elbow.

◆ CHAPTER ◆

14

The Foot and Ankle

Functionally as well as figuratively, the feet are a crucial part of our anatomy. An explorer proudly reports "setting foot" on undiscovered territory. We stamp our foot in anger, we impress others by "putting our best foot forward," we honor our teachers by "sitting at their feet," and we affirm independence by standing "on our own feet." Less poetically, the foot anchors us to earth and is highly adaptable to activity demands.

Anatomy of the Foot

One of the most remarkable aspects of evolution is that humans walk erect and that the two small feet support the body's entire weight. The superb architecture of the foot accounts for this feat.

The Bony Structures

Anatomically the foot has the same overall structure as the hand. Its twenty-six bones are subdivided into three groups: the *hindfoot,* the *midfoot,* and the *forefoot.*

The hindfoot consists of two bones: the *calcaneus,* or heel bone, and the *talus,* or ankle bone.

The midfoot consists of a collection of five irregularly shaped bones—the tarsal bones (or tarsus), which resemble the carpal bones of the wrist except that they are much larger. The tarsal bones include the navicular, the cuboid, and the three cuneiform bones. Collectively these bones function like ball bearings, promoting the rolling motion of the foot.

The forefoot consists of five rays, ending in the toes. Four of the rays have four bones; one, the big toe, also called *hallux*, consists of only three. The first and longest bone of each ray is called the metarsus, followed by the three (two for the big toe) phalanges of the toes. As with the hand, the phalanges of the toes are called the proximal, middle, and distal phalanges, and the joints between them are the metatarsal phalangeal joints and the proximal and distal phalangeal joints. The joints of the toes fit together like balls and sockets. As with the hand, each phalanx has a head, a shaft, and a base.

To enable the foot to function properly, its bones form two arches: *the longitudinal arch* and *the transverse arch*. These structures function like springs: they flatten when loaded and "spring back" to their original size when released. Sometimes these arches collapse, and the person is said to be flat-footed. The arches take time to develop, so young children are all flat-footed. Sometimes the arches don't develop at all, and this is congenital. In other words, you are born that way, and there is nothing much to do about it. On rare occasions, flat feet are the result of a gradual tearing of a supporting tendon, or a tightness of the heel (Achilles) cord. If the foot gradually becomes flat in adulthood it can become painful. Wearing arch supports corrects the condition temporarily. Flat feet, as a rule, do not lead to arthritis.

The Soft Tissues

Muscles, Ligaments, and Tendons

The bones of the foot are connected via countless ligaments. A crucial connector is the *Achilles tendon,* which runs from the calf muscle along the back of the heel. The Achilles tendon is the largest tendon in the entire body.

The Sole of the Foot (Plantar Surface)

From the bottom up, the metatarsal and tarsal bones of the foot form a triangular base that supports the weight of the body and helps maintain its balance.

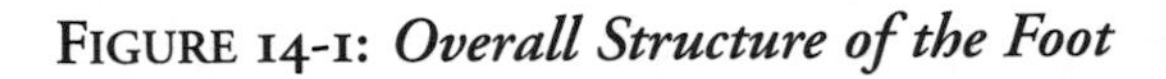

FIGURE 14-1: *Overall Structure of the Foot*

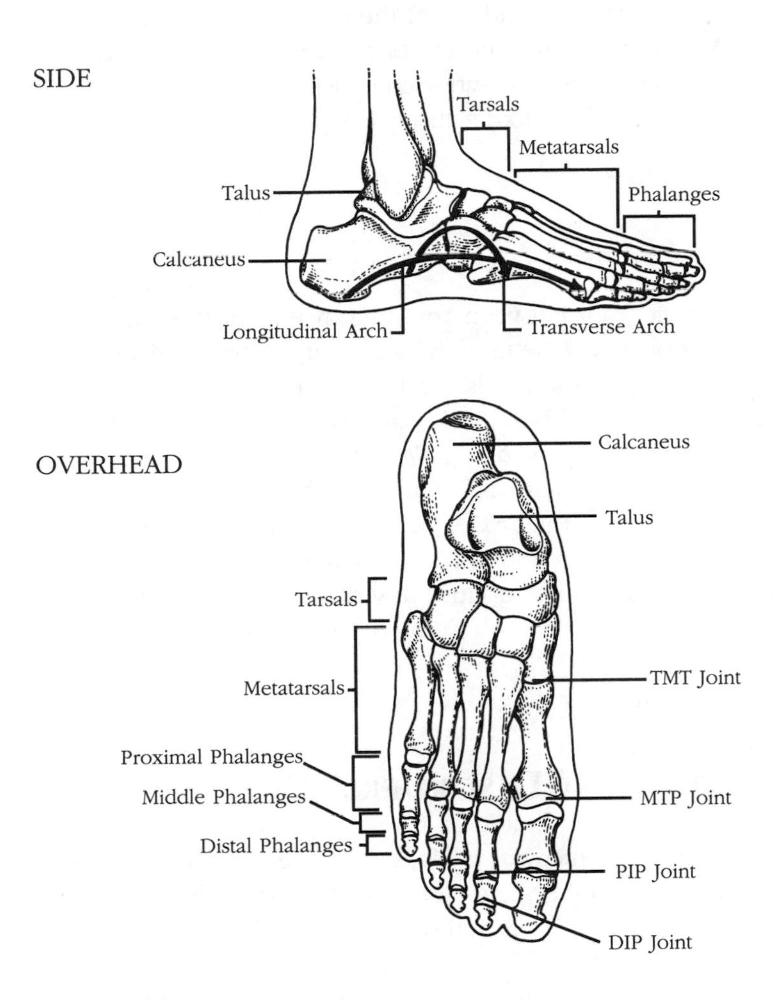

The foot is divided into the hindfoot (calcaneus and talus), midfoot (tarsal bones), and forefoot. Like the hand, the foot consists of a group of five "rays" of longitudinal bones that terminate in the toes. The midfoot consists of small bones that act as a ball bearing. The bones of the midfoot are arranged into two arches, the longitudinal arch and the transverse arch. Both flatten when compressed by the weight of the body and "spring back" when released.

Among the layers of soft tissue that form the underside of the foot is the thick *plantar fascia,* a band of connective tissue that issues from the *calcaneus* (heel bone), fans out, and inserts itself into some of the joints of the toes and various tendons of the feet. Chronic injury of the plantar fascia, often as a consequence of flat feet or overuse, causes some of the more common pain syndromes of the foot and especially the heel. Such foot pain feels like arthritis but is not.

The Ankle

The ankle is a hinge joint between the bottom end of the shin bone (tibia) and of the fibula and the talus. The prominent outer knob of the ankle is the lower end of the fibula, and the inner knob is the end of the tibia. Strong ligaments (the anterior and posterior *talofibular* ligaments and the *calcaneofibular and deltoid* ligaments) run from these knobs to the talus or calcaneus. Injury often stretches and tears ("sprains") the ligaments of the ankle. Depending on the position of the foot, one or more of these tendons can be damaged.

The ankle joint only moves up and down and does not rotate. The other movements of the foot, such as rotation or tilting, are provided by other structures.

Who Treats Foot Disorders?

For a very long time the medical profession neglected feet. This was unfortunate because several systemic diseases (i.e., disorders involving the entire body, including the internal organs) affect the feet. The joints of the feet are the first affected in 10 to 20 percent patients suffering from inflammatory arthritis. Therefore, it is important to consult a general internist, podiatrist, or orthopedic surgeon when you suffer from newly painful feet.

Podiatrists are specialists in diagnosing and treating diseases of the feet. They undergo a four-year-long training at special colleges of podiatry. Podiatrists are licensed to prescribe medications and perform limited surgery. To provide comprehensive foot care, many podiatrists work closely with physicians.

Who Has Osteoarthritis of the Feet?

According to a National Health Survey, 20 percent of the population between eighteen and seventy-nine years of age have evidence of osteoarthritis of the feet. The incidence increases with age. Between the ages of seventy-five and seventy-nine, about 50 percent of men and women show evidence of osteoarthritis. In this age group the arthritis was likely to be three times as severe in women than in men.

As usual, the presence of osteoarthritis does not always result in clinically symptomatic disease. In fact, primary, overt osteoarthritis of the feet is rare. Foot pain resulting from a combination of factors, including OA, ill-fitting shoes, minor injuries, and simply a lifetime of wear and tear is, however, very common and debilitating. The importance of keeping one's feet in good working order cannot be overemphasized for anyone suffering from degenerative joint disease of the hips, knees, or lower back. Therefore, in addition to other information, this chapter provides tips on selecting proper footwear.

Foot Disorders

Ruth J., now seventy-three years old, can't remember when she did not have trouble with her feet. At a very young age Ruth became a dental technician, spending hours on her feet. When she was twenty-five, a podiatrist prescribed orthotics (metal and leather shoe inlays), and that helped for a while.

In her late twenties Ruth quit work, raised her two daughters, kept an impeccable house, gardened, camped, and hiked with her family. Her feet, with their bunions and hammer toes, looked terrible, like those of a very old woman. But they were functional—at least until one Sunday back in 1985, when she took a long walk in the snow. After a while her feet hurt so much that she barely made it home. Early Monday morning she went to see an orthopedic surgeon.

◆ ◆ ◆ ◆ ◆ ◆ ◆

Disorders affecting the feet are so numerous that this chapter reviews only a few. In general, the healthy foot is so perfectly engineered that any disturbance—such as pain in or deformity of one of the toes—

affects overall function. Likewise, malposition of one of the toes very rapidly affects the others.

Disorders affecting the feet are subdivided into those affecting the forefoot, the midfoot, and the hindfoot. The most prevalent of the disorders affecting the forefoot involve the big toe and the second toe. Those affecting the hind foot involve a painful heel.

Bunions (Hallux valgus)

Most lay persons are familiar with bunions, the well-known knobs forming at the base of the big toe. This common foot disorder occurs when the phalanges of the big toe turn outward at the metatarsal joint. As a result the metatarsal bone forms an angle with the proximal phalanx. This often results in a painful swelling over the joint—a bunion. The medical name for bunion is hallux valgus.

Hallux valgus occurs much more often in women than in men. The initiating cause is not known, but genetic predisposition and prolonged wearing of inappropriate, pointy shoes are probably important contributing factors. Once started, the disease often progresses and may result in osteoarthritis. As the big toe moves outward it affects the alignment of the other toes. The second toe may be pushed upward or downward, or may become permanently bent, resulting in a hammer toe.

Medical Treatment

You might be able to live comfortably with your bunion(s) by shielding your big toe from additional pressure—for instance, wearing loose-fitting shoes or sandals. A special toe pad or custom-made orthotics may help. Treatment often involves NSAIDs.

Surgical Treatment

After all nonoperative measures failed, Ruth and her physician opted for surgery. That there are many different techniques for the surgical correction of hallux valgus deformity is one sure indication that surgical results are not always satisfactory. In Ruth's case the doctor removed the enlarged portion of the bone and the damaged portion of the metatarsal head. He also shortened the proximal phalanx and realigned the muscle's tendons and ligaments.

Recovery from foot surgery can be extremely long. It is never the goal to allow patients to wear pointy shoes, but to have them walk without pain in "normal" shoes.

Heel Spurs, Heel Pain

An excruciating painful heel is almost as familiar as bunions. For all intents and purposes a heel spur feels as if one were walking on a bruised heel or a sharp, splinterlike sliver of bone.

Actually, the cause of the pain is often the previously encountered plantar fascia—the thick band of connective tissue going from the heel to the sides of the foot and the toes—which may become overly stretched and calcified, resulting in what looks like a thorn or spur. The most common medical name for heel spur is *plantar fasciitis*—the ending *itis* meaning inflammation—in this case inflammation of this band of connective tissue. Related conditions include heel bursitis, painful fat pad syndrome, fat pad thinning, arthritis, vitamin deficiency, a tight Achilles tendon, and nerve entrapment ("pinched nerve") about the heel.

A stress fracture of the *calcaneus* (heel bone) can also present as heel pain. It can be particularly difficult to diagnose, as X rays often do not show these faint fractures. The condition is likely to occur in athletic people whose feet are repeatedly pounded by running.

Heel pain is usually well localized. It can be sharp or dull and is triggered by weight bearing while standing or walking. The pain is at its worst after one gets up in the morning or after a prolonged rest and also increases throughout the day.

Since heel pain can be a symptom of several serious disorders, its cause must be carefully investigated.

Medical Treatment

Though complete recovery takes months, nonsurgical treatment of heel spurs is successful in most cases. As usual, the first and most often effective treatment involves NSAIDs coupled with exercises. These include stretching of the Achilles tendon by bending the foot upwards.

A common regimen is repeated stretches (three to ten), held for ten seconds, three times a day. Athletes with heel spur syndrome should decrease the offending activity. All exercises should be done in moderation.

Heel cups or inlays, so fashioned that they protect the spur from impact, usually provide relief. Orthotics are usually custom-made by a skilled podiatrist or orthotist.

Patients who do not respond to the orthotics may respond to a local injection of anesthetic and corticosteroids. Surgery is a possibility for a selected few patients whose debilitating heel pain exceeds six months to one year, but it is rarely indicated.

Hallux Rigidus

Typical osteoarthritic bony proliferation can occur in the metatarsophalangeal joint (large joint) of the big toe. This results in pain and rigidity of the big toe, known as hallux rigidus. The condition must be differentiated from gout, which also frequently involves this same joint. In the case of *hallux rigidus,* an X ray will show typical degeneration of the joint.

Mild and moderate cases of *hallux rigidus* may respond to rest, anti-inflammatory medication, and proper shoes (with pads, supports, etc.) If none of these medical measures help, surgery may be indicated. Available procedures include debridement (removal of the bony spurs), resection of the joint, fusion of the metatarsophalangeal joint, or insertion of a plastic spacer.

Hammer Toe

Sometimes a toe—usually the one adjoining the big toe—curls up like a claw. Hammer toes can be congenital, but most often they develop because of inappropriate footwear or are secondary to a bunion deformity. Treatment of hammer toes involves manipulation, splinting, the use of felt pads, or surgical realignment.

Remember, most foot pain is preventable and treatable through proper footwear.

The Importance of Well-Fitting Shoes

Since so many painful foot problems are initiated by inappropriate footwear, let us briefly review what is meant by a well-fitting shoe. Humans have always fashioned shoes to protect their feet from injury.

Indeed, the primary purpose of shoes is to protect the feet, and today's hard pavement and unyielding floors magnify this need.

A good shoe must also provide support, cushion the foot, even out the distribution of forces, and allow the toes plenty of room. Some women's dress shoes, those with narrow toes and high heels, do not follow these principles. The pointed toe of the shoe crowds the toes by forcing them into an unnatural, triangular shape. High heels magnify this effect by shifting the weight of the body to the forefoot.

Ill-fitting footwear often result, over the long term, in foot deformities. The advent of sneakers and walking shoes is a welcome, healthy development. One cannot underestimate the importance of well-fitting shoes.

How to Select Well-Fitting Shoes

Well-fitting shoes are a must for all patients suffering from arthritis. Here are some pointers for selecting properly fitting shoes. Most of the suggestions come from The American Academy of Orthopaedic Surgeons patient education brochure called "Shoes, 100M193":

- Most people's right and left feet are of slightly different size. Feet also expand when bearing weight. Have the salesperson measure the length and width of each foot *while you stand,* and have the shoes fitted to the longer and wider foot. If necessary, use an insole in the shoe for the smaller foot.
- Feet swell during the day. Do not have your feet measured in the morning.
- The shoes you buy should be neither too large nor too small. Shoes that are too spacious offer too little support and may cause corns or blisters.
- Shoes should fit properly both at the toes and at the heels. Check to make sure your heel does not slip out. This is often a problem with nonlaced shoes. A shoemaker can sometimes narrow a heel by pasting material in the heel portion of the shoe.
- Don't select shoes by size alone. A certain size may be smaller or larger in another brand or style. Walk around in the shoes to make sure they fit well and feel comfortable. Do not buy shoes

that feel uncomfortable. There is no such thing as a "break-in period." With time, a foot may push or stretch a shoe to fit, but this can cause foot pain and damage.

- Be aware that shoe size may change as you age.
- For women, low-heeled shoes (one inch or lower) with a wide toe box (the front end of the shoe) are ideal.

◆ APPENDIX ◆

I

Common Questions Related to Osteoarthritis, Arthritis, and Other Musculoskeletal Disorders

Arthritis is often used as a catchall term for all disorders associated with joint and muscle pain. The following questions and answers provide additional facts on confusing issues, clarify obscure points, summarize information, define related musculoskeletal disorders, and address some topics not covered in this guide.

The assorted information is subdivided as follows:

Professionals Participating in Arthritis Care

Special Orthopedic Problems or Complications

Diagnostic Tests

Osteoarthritis and Related Musculoskeletal Disorders

General Questions

Living More Comfortably with Osteoarthritis

Medications

Surgery, Anesthesia, and Related Subjects

PROFESSIONALS PARTICIPATING IN ARTHRITIS CARE

What is an orthopedist?

An orthopedist is a physician and surgeon specializing in the treatment of musculoskeletal disorders, which include the muscle and joint problems discussed in this book. All orthopedists will choose among operative and nonoperative means to heal their patients.

What is the difference between a physical therapist (PT) and an occupational therapist (OT)?

Both play an important role in the treatment of osteoarthritis and in pain management. Their goal is to help arthritis patients lead more comfortable lives. Their approach to the patient is, however, different.

In general, physical therapists deal with large muscles and gross motor function, whereas occupational therapists concentrate on fine motor function.

Physical therapists teach range-of-motion exercises designed to maintain or increase joint mobility and strengthening exercises that rehabilitate the muscles surrounding the joints. They develop personal exercise programs adapted to each patient's needs, to be performed at home after discharge from the hospital. Physical therapists also teach good posture. If you need to use a cane, they make sure that it is properly adjusted to your height and that you use it correctly.

Physical therapists are skilled in providing pain relief with heat (hot packs, ultrasound, diathermy), transcutaneous nerve stimulation (TENS), or cold (ice packs). (See also Chapter 6, "Rehabilitation and Pain Management.")

A patient undergoing joint surgery may be evaluated by a physical therapist before the operation to determine whether special preoperative or postoperative care is needed. The skill of the physical therapist is essential once your joint has been operated on. Depending on the exact nature of the surgery, they might teach you how to get out of bed, sit in a chair, walk with a walker, or use crutches. They will help you eliminate fears about using your newly repaired joint and build up your confidence by providing successful movement experiences.

Occupational therapists are trained to help you carry on with your life in spite of arthritis. They are specialists in joint protection, and will teach you to maximize the pain-free use of your joints.

Occupational therapists are problem solvers. After evaluating your performance and your home environment, they are usually able to figure out ways in which you can carry out tasks that have become cumbersome or painful, such as cooking, writing, typing, combing your hair, eating, or driving. If indicated, occupational therapists may make splints to protect certain joints, especially the hand and wrists. (See also Chapter 13, "The Hand, Wrist, and Elbow.")

Occupational therapists will help you adapt your home and work environment to your specific needs, and they can recommend many useful devices, tools, and strategies to improve the quality of your life.

What is a chiropractor?

Chiropractic originated in the United States at the end of the nineteenth century. It is a therapeutic system based on the belief that diseases, in particular those related to the back, may be caused by abnormal functioning of the nervous system and may be relieved by appropriate manipulation of the spine. Chiropractors undergo training at accredited chiropractic colleges. Like other health professionals, chiropractors cannot alter the course of OA, but they may be able to temporarily alleviate pain.

What is an osteopath?

Osteopathy is an alternate school of medicine founded in 1874 by Dr. Andrew Taylor Still. Osteopaths believe that a disturbance in one physiological system affects the function of the entire body. Treatment is aimed at restoring equilibrium by traditional medical procedures (drugs, surgery, other) as well as physical manipulation. A Doctor of Osteopathy (DO) is a full-fledged physician qualified to practice all types of medicine and surgery. Like other health professionals, osteopaths cannot alter the course of OA, but they may be able to relieve the pain associated with the disease.

What is a podiatrist?

Podiatrists specialize in the diagnosis and treatment of diseases of the feet. Podiatrists undergo a four-year-long training at special colleges of podiatry and are licensed to prescribe medications and perform surgery such as reconstruction and fusion of toe joints.

Podiatrists are experts at fashioning orthotics—shoe inserts that can relieve foot and leg pain. Podiatrists are good at relieving pain associated with OA of the foot.

What is the function of the patient relations department?

Many hospitals have patient relations departments staffed by social workers or nurses who try to help patients with problems that may arise during their care. Such problems may concern medical billing, dealing with insurance companies, or complaints about hospital staff or fellow patients. If necessary, the patient relations department will arrange for counseling, transport by ambulette, home help, and stays in rehabilitation centers or nursing homes.

Special Orthopedic Problems or Complications

What is a "failed back"?

A failed back is persistent back pain after back surgery. As with any back dysfunction, the back pain is carefully evaluated, and appropriate treatment is instituted.

What is a "locked knee"?

A locked knee can't straighten because it is mechanically stuck. It is often caused by something broken or out of place within the knee. A free-floating fragment is one common cause for a locked knee. In this case, treatment involves removal of the loose body. Most often, however, locking is actually pseudolocking, which is caused by severe knee pain; this usually responds to Novocain.

What is a "non-union"?

Many orthopedic procedures, such as bunion surgery or leg realignment, involve cutting bone with fine instruments—the premise being that the bone will heal in its improved position. Occasionally, the body doesn't cooperate and the bone doesn't heal. Further surgery, electric stimulation, or the wearing of a cast are required to correct the situation. Non-union can also occur after a bone fracture (arm, leg, hip).

DIAGNOSTIC TESTS

Is there a blood test for osteoarthritis?

As yet there is no blood test to diagnose osteoarthritis. Scientists are trying to develop a test that identifies the debris released by an osteoarthritic joint. When such a test becomes available, doctors will be able to complete a diagnosis and start treatment before the osteoarthritis has caused much damage.

What is the difference between X rays, computerized axial tomography (CT scan), and magnetic resonance imaging (MRI)?

X-ray scans or pictures are relatively inexpensive and provide an adequate image of bones. Newer imaging techniques produce sharper, three-dimensional images. Computerized axial tomography (CT scan) is particularly good in providing details of bony tissue. Magnetic Resonance Imaging (MRI), which is even more expensive than a CT scan, provides good images of soft tissue. Very often a simple, old-fashioned X ray will provide sufficient diagnostic information. (For additional details see Chapter 11, "The Back and Neck.")

Osteoarthritis and Related Musculo-Skeletal Disorders

Is osteoarthritis hereditary?

Except for osteoarthritis of the fingers (Heberden's Nodes, see Chapter 13, "The Hand, Wrist, and Elbow") osteoarthritis is not usually hereditary.

Is the immune system involved in osteoarthritis?

No, the immune system does not malfunction in osteoarthritis. Remember, osteoarthritis affects one or more joints, not the body as a whole.

What is the difference between osteoarthritis and rheumatoid arthritis?

Rheumatoid arthritis is a systemic disease that affects the whole body and is associated with a malfunction of the immune system. It is often progressive, although it can go into spontaneous remission and disappear for months or years. Rheumatoid arthritis usually affects young adults. Since both diseases affect the joints, the surgical interventions discussed here are often used for patients suffering from rheumatoid arthritis as well as for those with osteoarthritis.

Can I have both osteoarthritis and rheumatoid arthritis?

Yes, occasionally. When this happens, the more complex and usually more severe rheumatoid arthritis supersedes the osteoarthritis.

Does osteoarthritis ever go away on its own?

No, the osteoarthritic changes that affect the joints are permanent. Don't despair. Many of the strategies suggested here—especially exercise, weight loss, and minor lifestyle changes—can help you overcome the limitations imposed by the disease.

What is osteoarthritis of the temporomandibular joint?

The two temporomandibular joints (TMJs) connect the mandible (jawbone) and the temporal bone at the base of the skull. These joints are occasionally affected by osteoarthritis, though dysfunction of the TM joint most often has other causes such as spasms of the chewing muscles or dental malocclusion (incorrect bite). Osteoarthritis of the TM joint is treated with local heat application, nonsteroidal anti-inflammatory drugs, and, if necessary, joint replacement surgery.

What is carpal tunnel syndrome (CTS)?

The carpal tunnel is a bony passage through the wrist bones, or "carpals." The median nerve, which carries messages to and from the thumb and certain fingers, passes from the arm to the hand through the tunnel. Carpal tunnel syndrome occurs when the tissues around the tunnel swell and compress the median nerve. Common symptoms of the syndrome are pain, numbness, and tingling. Later symptoms include muscle wasting, which may cause the sufferer to drop objects.

Carpal tunnel syndrome occurs most commonly in women at a time of hormonal change such as pregnancy or menopause, and in persons who must perform repetitive hand movements. The ailment is common among computer operators, including students, professionals, and supermarket clerks, as well as assembly-line workers.

Treatment involves splinting (especially during the night), NSAIDs, and possibly a corticosteroid injection. Surgical intervention (decompression) to relieve the pressure on the nerve may be necessary if the pain persists. Carpal tunnel syndrome is not related to arthritis.

What is chondromalacia patellae?

Chondromalacia is derived from the Greek words for cartilage (*chondros*) and softness (*malakia*). It is the term traditionally used to describe pain coming from the kneecap (patella), though softening is not always present. Often the condition is related to malalignment of the kneecap and/or damage to the cartilage in back of the kneecap. Chondromalacia patellae occurs most often, but not exclusively, in teenagers and young adults. Diagnosing the exact cause of the problem is important. Treatment consists of mild analgesics (aspirin,

NSAIDs, Tylenol), bracing, activity modification, and physical therapy. Surgery may be necessary in some cases. Chondromalacia patellae is not a rheumatic disease, but can occasionally result in OA.

What is fibromyalgia (fibrositis)?

Fibromyalgia, also called fibrositis, is a syndrome characterized by a combination of stiffness, muscle pain, overall aching in and around joints in various parts of the body, and fatigue. Symptoms are often so varied and vague that for very many years patients were often told that the syndrome was "all in their head." This is not the case. Fibromyalgia, like osteoarthritis, is a real disease. The discomfort of fibromyalgia often results from a vicious cycle of stress → muscle spasms → pain and tenderness → emotional stress.

The source of this pain comes from the muscles and from the points (trigger points) at which ligaments attach to muscles and bones.

Fibromyalgia improves with a restful, pleasurable lifestyle and is aggravated by stress. NSAIDs and other non-narcotic painkillers may help, as do muscle relaxants and sedatives. Another approach is to inject corticosteroids and local anesthetics into certain trigger points. Physical therapy, which teaches patients to spare certain vulnerable portions of their body, is helpful. Fibromyalgia commonly affects women between thirty and sixty years of age. Fibromyalgia is not related to arthritis.

What is giant cell arteritis?

See polymyalgia rheumatica (PMR) below.

What is osteomyelitis?

Osteomyelitis is infection of the bone and bone marrow usually by bacteria. As a rule, acute osteomyelitis responds to antibiotic treatment. Chronic osteomyelitis may require surgical excision of the affected bone as well as antibiotic therapy.

What is osteoporosis, and how does it differ from osteoarthritis?

Osteoporosis involves bones, and osteoarthritis involves the ends of bones, i.e., the joints. Osteoporosis involves bone thinning, and osteoarthritis often involves extra bone formation.

As discussed in Chapter 3, bone is constantly remodeled. As we age, bone loss exceeds bone replacement, and there is an overall loss of skeletal mass. In osteoporosis each bone element is mechanically and biochemically normal—there is just less of it. An osteoporotic bone often becomes very brittle and fractures readily. Hips are a good example. Statistical studies in the U.S. show that one woman in five will fracture her hip joint before her death. Interestingly, patients with osteoarthritis of the hip usually do not sustain hip fractures, even though osteoporosis and osteoarthritis are theoretically independent diseases.

Osteoporosis, like osteoarthritis, occurs more frequently in women than in men. The process is especially marked in women after menopause.

What is osteomalacia?

In osteomalacia there is inadequate mineralization or calcification of bone. The bone is therefore softer. Ostcomalacia can be the result of a number of disorders, many of which center on the metabolism of vitamin D. It is difficult to distinguish osteomalacia from osteoporosis by traditional X rays, although that differentiation is important because osteomalacia is often more treatable than osteoporosis. A biopsy is required to make a correct diagnosis.

What is polymyalgia rheumatica?

Polymyalgia rheumatica (PMR) is a painful arthritic condition characterized by muscle inflammation and stiffness. Treatment involves aspirin and other NSAIDs as well as corticosteroids. Polymyalgia rheumatica is self-limiting and goes away on its own within a matter of months or a few years. The condition primarily affects persons fifty years of age or older.

Giant cell arteritis (inflammation of the large blood vessel) is a common complication of PMR that, if untreated, may result in loss of vision. Warning signs of giant cell arteritis are headaches or pain and swelling of blood vessels near the temples. Fortunately, giant cell arteritis is one of the few rheumatic diseases that can be adequately and successfully treated by steroids.

What are polymyositis and dermatomyositis?

In these two connective tissue disorders the inflammation primarily affects muscle tissue. The disease may affect certain selected groups of muscles, such as those of the upper extremities or of the pelvis. Patients feel very weak—so weak that they may even have trouble combing their hair or getting out of bed. Fever, weight loss, and general malaise can occur.

In addition to these symptoms, patients suffering from dermatomyositis may have red, patchy skin rashes. (Remember that the skin, too, consists of connective tissue.) Treatment is highly individualized but usually includes corticosteroids, rest, and exercise.

General Questions

Is there a special diet for osteoarthritis?

No, unfortunately not, although some people say they feel better when they avoid nightshade vegetables like potatoes, eggplants, and tomatoes. However, because being overweight stresses the joints, diet nevertheless plays a crucial role in the treatment of osteoarthritis. It is essential to maintain a reasonable body weight.

Are alternative therapies bad?

Whenever medicine does not have all the answers concerning a particular disease, especially a chronic, painful one like arthritis, alternative treatments flourish. Many people with osteoarthritis have been told of the miraculous effects of a special diet, copper bracelets, moon dust, Chinese herb teas, or magic mud baths. There is nothing wrong with some of these unproven remedies except for the following:

- Unproven remedies are expensive. Based on a survey by the National Research Council, the Arthritis Foundation estimates that Americans spend a minimum of $1 billion annually on unproven remedies.
- A few unproven remedies are dangerous. (In a few cases some of the herb teas recommended for arthritis contained Butazolidin or Valium and have proved fatal.)
- Many of these remedies cause patients to delay seeking appropriate medical attention.

As with traditional medicine, use your common sense when evaluating alternative therapies.

What are orthotics?

Orthotics are shoe inserts designed to solve certain problems associated with walking. Most commonly orthotics are used to provide support for flat feet or relieve the pain of heel spurs. Under very special circumstances they may relieve knee pain. Orthotics are usually custom-made from cork, leather, or Plastozote. Orthotics are usually prescribed by an internist, orthopedist, or podiatrist.

Living More Comfortably with Osteoarthritis

How can I get into my car more easily?

People suffering from osteoarthritis of the hips or knees often have trouble getting in and out of cars. Here is how to do it more simply:

- Instead of getting into the car feet first, turn so that your back is to the seat; then sit and swing your legs into the car.
- Reverse the procedure to get out. Swing your feet out, rotating your body until you face the car door opening. Put your feet together on the ground and then stand.

My arthritic hands make it difficult for me to drive a car, peel potatoes, or hold a book. Any suggestions?

Your hands can do most of the things they've always done provided that the handles of the tools you use (peelers, knives, forks) are nice and fat. Leather automobile wheel covers make the steering wheel easier to grasp securely. You can order attachable handles, covers, and other tools through several mail order companies. The Arthritis Foundation's *Guide to Independent Living* lists many of these sources and makes thousands of suggestions on how to do most things.

Will a warm or dry climate help my osteoarthritis?

Cold, wet weather does not cause arthritis, but people suffering from arthritis usually feel better in warm weather. We would not advise you to move away from your family and friends just to live in a warm climate. Breaking up a long winter by taking a warm-weather vacation, however, is helpful.

Will a stay at a spa be good for my osteoarthritis?

A stay at a spa—with its warm water, exercise programs, massages, mud baths, and pampering—is wonderfully relaxing. It does not cure osteoarthritis, but most people who go feel better—for a while at least—after they come back.

What is the ideal pool temperature for swimming?

People suffering from osteoarthritis feel better in a warm pool than a cool one. About 83° is near ideal, but one often does not have a choice. Remember, even if the pool feels a bit cold when you enter it, you will usually start feeling comfortable once you start swimming. Wearing a swim cap can make the water feel warmer.

MEDICATIONS

I have taken aspirin for more than five years. Should I worry about long-term effects?

As with any medication, aspirin may have long-term effects, and if you take aspirin regularly, you should discuss this with your doctor. However, the most common side effect of aspirin is stomach irritation. If this happens, you might consider discontinuing its use, or taking it along with a medication that protects the lining of your stomach. You may also be able to switch to Tylenol (acetaminophen), which does not irritate the stomach.

Is sustained-release aspirin better than regular aspirin?

The body gets rid of aspirin very quickly. To be effective aspirin must thus be taken very frequently. Aspirin formulated as a sustained-release formulation is so engineered that additional medication is released at predetermined time intervals. This type of pill has to be taken less often than standard aspirin.

Does aspirin interfere with my anticoagulant (blood thinning) medication?

Yes. Aspirin is an anticoagulant and augments the action of your prescription anticoagulant. Check with your doctor if you take aspirin and/or an anticoagulant regularly.

What about the new over-the-counter painkillers advertised on television?

Aspirin and acetaminophen were discovered a long time ago, long before there were government agencies regulating the sale of medications. That is why these two drugs are available without prescription. Recently the pharmaceutical industry has developed about twenty aspirinlike drugs, such as Indocin, Motrin, Naproxen, and Feldene. These nonsteroidal anti-inflammatory drugs (NSAIDs) are gentler on the stomach than aspirin. Two of these NSAIDs are available without prescription: ibuprofen (Motrin-IB, Advil, Nuprin, Rufen, and others) and naproxen (Aleve).

Are steroids ever used for osteoarthritis?

Corticosteroids are never taken in pill form for osteoarthritis. Occasionally corticosteroids are injected into a specific joint to temporarily relieve pain. Sometimes such pain relief, which lasts for two to three months, enables the soft tissues of a joint to heal. For more details see Chapter 13, "The Hand, Wrist, and Elbow."

I have a total joint prosthesis. Why should I take antibiotics before going to the dentist or when I have certain diagnostic tests?

One of the most feared complications of total joint replacement is infection of the prosthesis. During dental work, and also during certain invasive diagnostic procedures, bacteria may enter your blood. Theoretically, these microorganisms may become lodged in your artificial joints, causing infection there. To reduce this small chance, physicians advise their patients to take antibiotics prophylactically before undergoing such procedures. (Some physicians question the need for antibiotic treatment prior to dental procedures.)

Surgery, Anesthesia, and Related Subjects

When is arthroscopy used?

The arthroscope (see Chapter 11) is a fiber-optic instrument that, after insertion, permits visualization of joint surfaces. This excellent diagnostic tool can be used to examine any joint in the body, even the temporomandibular joint, which connects the mandible (jaw bone) and the temporal bone of the skull.

The arthroscope is increasingly used for appropriate repair jobs in

ankles, to smooth out rough cartilage, remove bone spurs and loose bodies elbows, for similar problems

knees, to remove the torn portion(s) of the meniscus or loose bodies

shoulders, to repair the edges of torn tendons, remove loose bodies, or trim the acromium

wrists, to remove debris and smooth rough cartilage

How can I protect my total hip prosthesis?

The greatest dangers to your prosthesis are infection, dislocation, loosening, and wear.

Infection is minimized by taking prophylactic antibiotics when going to the dentist (see page 242) or undergoing certain diagnostic procedures. Dislocation is minimized by avoiding certain maneuvers. For example, avoid sitting in low chairs, which may position the knee above the operated hip. Loosening and wear are minimized by reducing stress as much as possible, avoiding sudden-impact activities such as jumping or running, and avoiding excessive weight gain.

How can I protect my total knee prosthesis?

As a rule, knee prostheses do not dislocate, but, as with hip prostheses, infection, loosening and wear can pose problems. Precautions are the same as those mentioned for the hip.

What is the difference between a cemented and a noncemented prosthesis?

Most prostheses are attached to bone using methylmethacrylate cement. Since this cement has a tendency to loosen after a number of years, doctors have developed prostheses with porous surfaces that permit the in-growth of the patient's own bone. Such noncemented prostheses take longer to heal and are not necessarily better than cemented prosthesis. Discuss the options with your physician.

How long do I stay in the hospital after a total joint replacement?

Length of stay varies from region to region and depends on the availability of step-down facilities for physical therapy and rehabilitation. Actually most patients are ready to leave the acute care setting within four or five days but may stay in the hospital for a week to ten days to work with rehabilitation specialists.

What is epidural anesthesia?

During epidural anesthesia, a local anesthetic is injected into in the epidural space (a padded layer surrounding and protecting the spinal cord) in the spinal column. An injection in the lower back numbs the nerves of the abdomen and legs.

What is the difference between local and regional anesthesia?

During local anesthesia, Lidocaine or another local anesthetic is injected into the portion of the body that is being operated on. During regional anesthesia, also called nerve block anesthesia, a local anesthetic is injected in a site whose nerves control the sensory path of the treated area. Administering anesthetics in this manner numbs an entire part of the body, usually an arm or a leg. For instance, during bunion surgery, Novocain is injected around the ankle, and the entire foot becomes numb. Novocain can be injected around the shoulder to make the entire arm numb.

What is an autologous blood transfusion?

It means that the blood you donate prior to surgery will be transfused back into your own body during or after the surgery. Donating your own blood avoids the very small danger of adverse reactions or disease being transmitted by blood transfusion. Autologous blood transfusion is less expensive than ordinary blood transfusion.

◆ APPENDIX ◆

II

A Fresh Look at the Treatment of Osteoarthritis

THE TREATMENT OF OSTEOARTHRITIS

Patients suffering from osteoarthritis who are looking for new methods of managing their disease can cautiously cheer: An increasing number of scientists are searching for drugs and other treatments that hopefully might protect cartilage from degradation. Such substances are referred to as chondroprotective (from the Greek chondro = cartilage).

The effectiveness of these experimental substances is difficult to evaluate because the damage caused by osteoarthritis is unpredictable and slow. In addition, the pain associated with osteoarthritis waxes and wanes. As discussed, in any clinical study concerning arthritis, thirty percent of all participants improve, regardless of whether they actually received the active pill or treatment or only believed they did. This is the so-called placebo effect.

Some of the newer treatments involve constituents related to normal cartilage, others pertain to new drugs, others still attempt to coax the cartilage into repairing itself. To understand the mechanisms scientists hope to utilize, let us briefly review the constitution of cartilage discussed extensively in Chapter 3.

The Constituents of Articular Cartilage

Articular cartilage consists of various fibrous proteins (collagens) and proteoglycans (formerly called mucopolysaccharides). The latter are long chains (polymers) of carbohydrates known as glycosaminoglycans—types of complex sugars containing sulfate and amino groups—which are linked to a protein core by specific chemical bonds. (The carbohydrate portion of the compounds accounts for 90 percent.) The most abundant of the proteoglycans are the chondroitin sulfate proteoglycans.

The proteoglycans are structured to carry a considerable electric charge that enables these compounds to absorb large quantities of water and act as biological lubricants and shock absorbers. The water content of intact cartilage renders it resilient.

Other biochemical substances closely related to the proteoglycans include heparin, a familiar anticoagulant (blood thinner), and the keratan sulfates of the cornea and other structural tissues.

Hyaluronan (formerly called hyaluronic acid) is another closely related body chemical. Hyaluronan again is a glycosaminoglycan (not linked to protein) that can bind large amounts of water. It functions as a lubricant and shock absorber. Hyaluronan is an essential constituent of synovial fluid as well as of the vitreous humor that fills the eye ball. A dramatic decrease in the viscosity of the synovial fluid is one of the hallmarks of most forms of arthritis, including osteoarthritis.

Are Glucosamine and Chondroitin Sulfate an Arthritis Cure?

Health food stores have been buzzing with activity. Their new clients are patients suffering from osteoarthritis and other forms of joint pain who buy vast quantities of glucosamine and chondroitin sulfate. These substances are said to cure arthritis.

Proponents of the miracle arthritis cure believe that the greater availability of cartilage building blocks would reduce the breakdown of the cartilage characteristic of osteoarthritis. The treatment has been used for several years in Europe as well as in veterinary medicine in this country. And there are a number of studies that indicate that patients taking from 750–1500mg glucosamine and chondroitin sulfate/day experience a definite reduction in joint pain, stiffness, and even a reduction in joint swelling.

Chondroitin sulfate and glucosamine are considered nutritional supplements, and, as such, their sale is not regulated by the Food and Drug Administration, and thus they are not certified as either safe or effective. They can be freely purchased. So far, fortunately, except for some occasional diarrhea, the two substances seem to be safe enough to take.

Arthritis specialists and biochemists are skeptical about whether these substances are incorporated into cartilage. Even though glucosamine and chondroitin sulfate are absorbed when taken by mouth, it is usually difficult to "convince" the adult body to utilize extra amounts of externally supplied raw material into its own tissue. For instance, no amount of calcium supplementation halted the progression of osteoporosis. (The discovery of Fozamax, a drug that slows the action of one of the enzymes involved in bone thinning, did the trick. Today Fozamax is widely prescribed, and osteoporosis has become treatable.)

Nevertheless since so many patients report feeling better on a regimen that includes glucosamine and chondroitin sulfate, some arthritis specialists are investigating their reports even though most believe that the success of these nutritional supplements is coincidental. Here are several explanations for the reported success of glucosamine and chondroitin sulfate:

- The author of *The Arthritis Cure*, Dr. Jason Theodosakis, recommends an effective exercise and weight loss program, similar to the ones recommended in *The Columbia-Presbyterian Osteoarthritis Handbook*. These measures, indeed, provide relief for most patients suffering from osteoarthritis.
- Chondroitin sulfate and glucosamine may cause pain relief, which would result in better mobility and reduced swelling.
- The substances may inhibit some of the enzymes that participate in the degradation of collagen.
- Anyone who suffers from arthritis knows that pain comes and goes, often without rhyme or reason. Arthritis patients blame the weather, swear by dietary modifications or even something as innocent as wearing copper bracelets. Psychological factors do play a role. As a rule, all patients feel better after they visit their doctor. And, as discussed, thirty percent of all patients improve on placebo.

Doyt Conn, M.D., the Medical Director of the Arthritis Foundation in Atlanta, believes that it is unlikely that the "Arthritis Cure" results in a permanent improvement. According to the Foundation, the European studies on which the hype is based were poorly controlled, and on the basis of currently available data, the Arthritis Foundation cannot advise people to take these preparations.

CHONDROPROTECTIVE AGENTS

Scientific attention is currently focusing on substances that will protect the joint by:

- Stimulating the formation of collagen, proteoglycans, and hyaluronan
- Inhibiting enzymes that degrade cartilage
- Suppress inflammation

Leading candidates include the polyproteoglycans.

A number of variants of the proteoglycan sulfates that are the major building blocks of cartilage have been tested.

Pentosan Polysulfate

Peter Ghosh, an Australian rheumatologist, has tried this synthetic polysulfate on patients suffering from osteoarthritis, animal models, and on tissue culture and has shown that it:

- Protects articular cartilage
- Stimulates the synthesis of hyaluronan
- Slows the degradation of cartilage

Clinical trials are now underway.

Two other closely related substances: Arteparon (glycosaminoglycan polysulfate) and Rheumalon (glycoaminoglycan peptide), had proven successful in clinical trials. These drugs had to be discontinued because of various side effects, thereby proving that one must exercise caution in trying new, unapproved therapies.

Hylans

Patients suffering from osteoarthritis fantasize about having their joints lubricated like the Tin Man, from the *Wizard of Oz*. Viscosupplementation of the synovial fluid appears to be one such alternative, though the substance injected actually does not remain for very long in the joint cavity.

Since joint dysfunction is usually associated with an alteration of the consistency of the synovial fluid, E. A. Balazs and his associates attempted to increase the viscosity of this body fluid. The obvious candidate was hyaluronan, a body chemical, tried thirty years ago on race horses with traumatic arthritis: After treatment the animals were able to train and race without disabling pain. After years of scientific investigation, Synvisc, a highly polymerized hyaluronan, with very high viscoelastic properties, was tried on humans. Indeed, three injections of Synvisc offers pain relief and improved joint function when injected into the knee joint.

Numerous clinical studies involving hundreds of patients, have proven the procedure relatively safe. In up to 84 percent of patients, pain relief and enhanced function lasted an average of eight months. Local adverse reactions were noted in 2–3 percent of patients.

The procedure is currently available in Canada and in many European countries. Treatment, so far, is restricted to the knee joint.

More About Drugs

Doxacycline

Kenneth Brandt, L.P. Yu Jr., and their colleagues at Indiana University have discovered that doxycycline, an antibiotic, is effective in inhibiting cartilage breakdown in animals. It is not yet known whether the antibiotic can reverse existing osteoarthritic lesions. The tests were so successful that the substance is now being tried in humans.

NSAIDS

Detailed investigation of the standard NSAIDS have shown that, as far as osteoarthritis is concerned, there is considerable difference between various agents. Some of the newer ones, notably diclofenac and piroxicam, affected cartilage metabolism favorably, while others were either indifferent and some even harmful.

COX-2 Inhibitors

Within the next few years the pharmaceutical industry will release an entirely new class of drugs called the COX-2 (short for cyclooxygenase, one of the enzymes of the prostaglandin cascade) inhibitors. For arthritis, these remarkable new drugs may supplant aspirin and its near relatives, the NSAIDS.

As discussed in Chapter 4, the NSAIDS work because they interfere with the hormone-like prostaglandins, substances that mediate pain and inflammation. Prostaglandins, however, also participate in the control of many other important biological functions and—as anyone who has taken these agents for a while knows—the NSAIDS have many unpleasant side effects, of which those affecting the gastrointestinal tract are the most bothersome. The COX-2 inhibitors interrupt the prostaglandin cascade at a later point in the cycle, thereby eliminating many of the objectionable side effects of the NSAIDS.

Gamma-Linolenic Acid as an Anti-Inflammatory

For a number of years the role of certain highly polyunsaturated fatty acids (PUFA) has been studied by a number of scientists. These fatty acids found in fish oils and plant seeds are the precursors of the hormone-like prostaglandins that play such an important role in many body processes (see above). Recently the anti inflammatory effects of gamma-linolenic acid, a PUFA, have been studied in animal models and in patients suffering from rheumatoid arthritis.

The small number of patients included in a double blind study had a statistically significant and encouraging decrease in pain, morning stiffness, and in the number of swollen and tender joints. Gamma-linolenic may turn out to be useful in the treatment of osteoarthritis whose inflammatory component is still being evaluated. Like chondroitin sulfate and glucosamine, PUFA's are considered nutritional supplements, and not drugs, and their sale is not regulated by the Food and Drug Administration.

Cartilage Cell Transplants

Initial experiments with cartilage cell transplants have led to some cautious optimism in the repair of traumatic knee injuries. In animal experiments, cartilage cells were harvested from a healthy joint and grown in tissue culture to form new cartilage. This cultured cartilage was then used to repair a joint with experimentally induced arthritis.

In humans, healthy cells obtained from the patient's healthy knee joint were again grown in tissue culture. Then the cells were reinjected in the injured knee joint, fostering its recovery. This still experimental procedure works best for patients with isolated cartilage defects and can only be used for younger patients. After age 50–55, cartilage cells no longer reproduce in tissue culture. But, at any age recovery is slow and requires the prolonged use of crutches.

◆ APPENDIX ◆

III

Nonsteroidal Anti-Inflammatory Drugs for the Treatment of Osteoarthritis

The following nonsteroidal anti-inflammatory drugs are currently used for the treatment of osteoarthritis. The term T ½ (half-life) refers to the number of hours it takes your body to get rid of half the drug. The body eliminates drugs with a short T ½ very quickly. Drugs that are eliminated slowly have a long T ½. A drug's half-life dictates how often it has to be taken.

For example, one dose a day will do for piroxicam (Feldene), which has a T ½ of fifty hours. On the other hand, for continuous pain relief one has to take six doses of aspirin (T ½ of only thirty minutes).

Nonsteroidal Anti-Inflammatory Drugs

Generic Name*	Trade Name**	T ½ hours approximate	Form/ Dosage
Acetylsalicylic acid	Aspirin, others	.5	Tablets: 325 mg 500 mg
Diclofenac	Voltaren	1–2	Tablets: 25 mg 50 mg 75 mg
COMMENT: Drug is enteric coated.			
Diflunisal	Dolobid	8–12	Tablets: 250 mg 500 mg
COMMENT: The drug is a salicylate like aspirin.			
Etolac	Lodine	7.3	Capsules: 200 mg 300 mg
Fenoprofen Calcium	Nalfon	3	Capsules: 200 mg 300 mg Tablets: 600 mg
COMMENT: Should not be used by patients suffering from kidney disease.			
Flurbiprofen	Ansaid	6	Tablets: 50 mg 100 mg
COMMENT: Maximum 300 mg/day.			

* **GENERIC NAME:** This is the common name of the drug.

** **TRADE NAME:** Also referred to as proprietary name, is the name given to the drug by the manufacturer. Sometimes, as in the case of aspirin, the trade name becomes so familiar that people use it as if it were the generic name. In reality, aspirin's generic name is acetylsalicylic acid. Most of the drugs listed here are available in Canada under different trade names.

Information in table form: *The Nurse's Drug Handbook*, seventh edition, by Suzanne Loebl, George R. Spratto, and Adrienne L. Woods (Delmar, 1994).

Generic Name	Trade Name	T ½ hours approximate	Form/ Dosage
Ibuprofen	Motrin	2	Tablets: 300 mg 400 mg 600 mg 800 mg
	Rufen	2	Tablets: 400 mg 600 mg 800 mg

COMMENT: This drug is available without prescription. All OTC products contain 200 mg per tablet. Other trade names of these preparations include Advil, Ibiprin, Ibu-Tab, Menadol, Midol 200, Nuprin, others.

Generic Name	Trade Name	T ½ hours approximate	Form/ Dosage
Indomethacin	Indocin	5	Capsules: 25 mg 50 mg Rectal Suppo-sitories: 50 mg
	Indocin SR	5	Capsules: 75 mg
Ketoprofen	Orudis	2–5	Tablets: 25 mg

COMMENT: Should be used at reduced dosage by the elderly and patients suffering from kidney disease.

Generic Name	Trade Name	T ½ hours approximate	Form/ Dosage
Ketorolac	Acolar, Toradol	4–6	Tablet: 10 mg Also available for IM injection
Meclofenamate sodium*	Heclofen, Meclomen	2–3	Tablets*: 50 mg 100 mg
Mefenamic Acid	Ponstel	2–4	Capsules: 250 mg

COMMENT: Use one week only.

Generic Name	Trade Name	T ½ hours approximate	Form/ Dosage
Mesalamine	Asacol	.5–1.5	Suppositories, Rectal Suspension Tablet, delayed release

COMMENT: Not indicated for patients with sensitivity to sulfite.

Generic Name	Trade Name	T ½ hours approximate	Form/ Dosage
Nabumetone	Relafen	22–30	Tablets: 500 mg 750 mg
Naproxen	Naprosyn	12–15	Tablets: 250 mg 375 mg 500 mg
Naproxen Sodium	Anaprox Sodium	12–13	Tablets: 250 mg 375 mg 500 mg

COMMENT: *This drug is available without prescription. The OTC product contains 200 mg per tablet. Other trade name: Aleve.*

Generic Name	Trade Name	T ½ hours approximate	Form/ Dosage
Oxaprozin	Daypro	20–25	Caplets: 600 mg
Phenylbutazone	Butazolidine, many others	72	Capsules: 100 mg Tablets: 100 mg

COMMENT: *This is another older drug that is seldom used, and then only for short periods of time, because it may cause serious blood disease (agranulocytosis).*

Generic Name	Trade Name	T ½ hours approximate	Form/ Dosage
Piroxicam	Feldene	50	Capsules: 10 mg 20 mg

COMMENT: *This drug is extremely long lasting (long half-life).*

Generic Name	Trade Name	T ½ hours approximate	Form/ Dosage
Sulindac	Clinoril	8	Tablets: 150 mg 200 mg
Tolmetin	Tolectin	1	Capsules: 400 mg Tablets: 400 mg

Glossary

Advanced Directives—Instruction "directing" medical care personnel to carry out your wishes about health care should you be unable to provide appropriate instructions. Similar to living will.

Analgesic—A medication that relieves pain.

Arthritis—The term, which literally means "joint inflammation," applies to a group of more than a hundred rheumatic diseases. These diseases can affect not only the joints but also other connective tissues in the body, including the muscles, tendons, ligaments, skin, and certain internal organs.

Arthroplasty—Reconstruction of any joint.

Arthroscope—A small, pencil-sized fiber-optic instrument used for both diagnosis and surgery.

Autologous Blood Transfusion—Donation of your own blood before a medical procedure in view of having this blood reinfused after surgery.

Biofeedback Training—A technique that enables you to control certain unconscious biological functions, such as pain and blood pressure, by means of a conscious thought process.

Bursa—Small, fluid-filled pouch of connective tissue that serves to cushion the joints.

Bouchard's Nodes—Bony nobs forming on the proximal interphalangeal joints of the fingers.

Bursitis—Inflammation of the small bursae that cushion the various components of a joint. The condition is often caused by excessive pressure on the joint. Common examples are "housemaid's knees," shoulder bursitis, and "student's elbows."

Cartilage—A tough, resilient tissue that covers and cushions the ends of the bones and absorbs shock.

Collagen—The main structural protein of skin, tendon, bone, cartilage, and connective tissue.

Computerized Axial Tomography (CT or CAT Scan)—An imaging technique that produces detailed three-dimensional images of soft tissues, including joints and inner organs.

Debridement—Surgical "cleansing" of a joint or wound to expose healthy tissue and promote healing. In the case of joints, debridement refers to removal of loose cartilage, foreign bodies, osteophytes, dead tissue, bone chips, and inflamed synovial tissue to reduce pain and improve function of joint.

Degenerative Joint Disease—Another name for osteoarthritis (OA).

Fibrous Capsule—A tough wrapping consisting of the tendons and ligaments that surround the joint.

Half-time—Related to the length of time a drug stays active in the blood.

Heberden's Nodes—Bony growths or spurs that form on the distal interphalangeal joints of the fingers.

Heel Spur—Calcification or spurs of the plantar facia, the tough connective tissue sheet running from the heel to the ball of the foot.

Ligament—Band of cordlike tissue that connects bone to bone.

Magnetic Resonance Imaging (MRI)—Diagnostic imaging technique that produces detailed, three-dimensional images of soft tissues, including the joints and internal organs, using electromagnets instead of X rays.

Methmethacrylate Cement—The bonding material surgeons use to anchor prostheses to bone.

Muscle—Tissue that has the ability to contract, producing movement of a joint.

Nonsteroidal Anti-Inflammatory Drugs (NSAIDs)—A group of drugs, such as aspirin or aspirinlike drugs, used to reduce the pain and inflammation characteristic of arthritis.

Orthotics—Corrective devices, such as inlays, heel cups, and toe spaces for shoes; designed to correct or relieve major and minor deformities of the feet.

Osteoarthritis—The rheumatic disease that affects cartilage, causing it to fray, wear, ulcerate, and in extreme cases, disappear entirely, leaving a joint in which bone rubs on bone. Disability results most often from disease in the weight-bearing joints (knees, hips, and spine).

Osteoblasts—Cells whose principal function is to form new bone.

Osteoclasts—Cells whose principal function is to resorb bone.

Osteophytes—Bony growths, usually trigged by an attempt by a traumatized or diseased joint to repair the frayed edge of the bone.

Osteoporosis—Disease characterized by demineralizaton of the skeleton resulting in bone loss and sometimes fractures.

Osteotomy—The surgical cutting of a bone.

Prostaglandin—A hormonelike regulator that governs many body processes including inflammation, kidney function, and gastric acid secretion.

Range of motion—The ability and degree to which a joint can move.

Recommended Daily Allowance (RDA)—Minimal amount of an essential nutrient a person should eat each day.

Spinal Fusion—Surgical procedure which removes the intervertebral disks and "fuses" adjacent vertebrae by filling in the empty spaces with bone grafts.

Spinal Stenosis—Narrowing of the opening through which the nerve roots exit from the spinal canal.

Synovectomy—Surgical removal of the synovium, the thin mucous-producing lining of the joint capsule.

Synovium—Thin lining of joint cavity that produces the synovial fluid that lubricates the joint.

Synovium—Cellophane-like tissue that lines the joint cavity. The synovium produces synovial fluid, which nourishes and lubricates the joints.

Systemic—Affecting the entire body, including the inner organs.

Tendinitis—Inflammation of a tendon connecting a particular bone with a particular muscle. Typical examples are "tennis elbow," "golfer's elbow," and tendinitis of the shoulder and the Achilles tendon in the heel.

Tendon—Fibrous cord that connects muscle to bone.

Transcutaneous Electric Nerve Stimulation (TENS)—Method of pain relief consisting of repeated small shocks of electricity. The method is believed to work by overloading and counterirritating pain transmission nerve paths.

Ultrasound—High-frequency sound waves used as heat treatment for musculoskeletal diseases.

Unproven Remedies—Treatments outside acceptable medical standards.

Index

A

B

C

D

E

F

G

H

I

J

K

L

M

N

O

P

Q

R

S

T

U

V

W

X

Y

Z